"I first started working wi Consulting about eleven boom; however, the boom settled shortly thereafter. And that's where Kelly and PGC were effective at helping physicians drive patients to their practices. Their events were amazing–averaging $60,000-$70,000 per event, and this was a time where most people had never heard of laser lipolysis.

"Fast forward 11 years later, they're working with us today on BodyTite and Votiva by InMode and they've been driving a tremendous number of patients to practices. We have extremely happy physicians that wanted to grow their practices but didn't know if the investment they were making was worthwhile. But with PGC, we have full confidence in their ability to help these doctors recoup their investment, making it extremely easy for us to work in a capital equipment world."

-Shakil Lakhani, President, North America, InMode

"Under Kelly Smith's direction, I have trusted the PGC team for the last decade to help practices get off to a fast start once they purchase a new medical device. They've been able to implement the controls necessary to ensure long-term success at these practices. I have been consistently impressed with their ability to help doctors increase revenue so quickly and make the process fluid no matter the location of the practice or types of services they offer. Kelly's program was one of the best kept secrets in aesthetics–now it is a must have for all aesthetic practices."

-Glenn Normoyle, Former President, NeoGraft Hair Transplantation

"Kelly Smith was referred to me by her accounting firm. When I met with her and discovered how successful she had been at not only growing her business revenue...she did it by helping other high end businesses grow their revenue. I meet with some of the most successful people in business and advise them on their personal and professional financial affairs. Kelly is the only client

I have ever asked to look at my own business. She has helped us create and implement a strategy which has helped us to grow our own revenue to a new high within the firm. There is no one I could recommend with higher confidence if someone wants to grow their bottom line. All while making it more efficient, fun, and solve those hard to face personality conflicts we all struggle with internally and with external customers as well. Want to win...I would meet with Kelly Smith."

-Brad Desormeau, Owner, The Northwest Wealth Consulting Group

"Never have I been so impressed by such a profound woman in the aesthetic world of business. I have worked with Kelly Smith for over 6 years while partnering with Projected Growth Consulting & Web.com. She has referred hundreds of clients to me for search engine marketing. Her processes, systems, and creative thinking work wonders for her clients' growth. I have seen practices transformed when they undergo her programs for patient acquisition and follow the team's advice. This book is an insight to all of her hard work in the industry, decades of financial experience, and in owning and operating businesses. Kelly and PGC will revolutionize how practices think about increasing revenue."

-Amber K. McCarter, Senior Sales Executive, Web.com

"Kelly is a creative and innovative thinker, which truly comes across when she shares her marketing and strategic insights. She has worked closely with top clients, delivering unprecedented practice results with passion. Her knowledge and expertise in the aesthetics industry is refreshing—helping practices build their businesses in a unique way. Practices face a multitude of obstacles when starting a new practice or navigating growth. The industry is better with individuals like Kelly who can guide a practice to success."

-Yang Phan, VP Marketing Operations, Invasix

"Experience was very positive from the beginning of planning the event with marketing and timeline, all the way to the actual presentation and patient discussion/questions and signups! Very helpful. Also, the presentation went very smoothly and patients really enjoyed the evening."

-Joshua Roller, MD, Arkansas
Event sales $216,000

"We had lots of questions and PGC was very patient, gracious and held our hand every step of the way! They did an excellent job credentialing our practice."

-Center for Reconstructive Surgery, Michigan
Event Sales $160,000

"From the time that we bought our machine, PGC has been partnering with us the whole time. They provided us with great communication, materials, and were very professional. We had a fun, interactive event. They've been totally amazing. I highly recommend them."

-Kris Shewmake, MD, Arkansas
Event Sales $160,000

"We needed someone to provide a fun welcoming experience for the patients to learn about our new device and it was definitely delivered. PGC was awesome! So professional, entertaining and informative! We were extremely pleased! The patients all commented on how much they enjoyed 'learning' about the procedure!"

-Stephen Gauthier, MD, Oklahoma
Event Sales $156,000

"As a new NeoGraft provider, we were a bit nervous about getting our first event scheduled. PGC far exceeded our expectations."

-Kevin Duplechain, MD, Louisiana
Event Sales $153,700

"We loved how PGC helped us streamline our event process. Helping us vet candidates, supplied excellent paperwork help, and really focused this experience for our patients in the most profitable way. They were simply the best!"

-Tiffany McCormack, MD, Nevada
Event Sales $137,480

"We had an awesome turnout. Almost 100% signed up tonight. We had awesome support from PGC. They created a great powerpoint, and used great before and after pictures. We're pumped, looking forward to the next month or two, and hoping to pay off our device."

-Scott Ferguson, MD, Florida
Event Sales $105,000

"I really appreciated the YouTube videos you had on having launch events and social media. Thank you for your advice, it was very helpful. My consultant was very enthusiastic and had a log of great ideas and tips."

-Lá-Shaun Elliott, MD, Hale Health Care, Woodstock, GA

"I have benefited from Kelly and her team's extensive knowledge of the business side of operating an aesthetics business. PGC has vast experience with various technologies, they can give me unbiased advice on what they have seen work in other offices. Additionally, I have worked with them for over a year running my social media for my office. It has been a great benefit to our growth and a weight off my team."

-Brian Stolley, MD, President, MediSpa Maui, Maui, HI

"Our work with Kelly Smith and the PGC Team has included launch events, sales and marketing and an ongoing social media and digital marketing relationship for one year. Their ability to guide us through converting insurance pay patients to cash for service clients has been a vital part of our growth and success."

-Scott T. Guenthner, MD, Plainfield, IL

"Excellent delivery of technology highlights. Helped secure multiple patient leads and procedures. Very friendly, approachable and professional. Overall excellent performance!"

-Jordan P. Sand, MD, Spokane, WA

"Working with Kelly and her team at PGC has been a truly positive experience for our Facial Plastic Surgery practice. PGC's team creates creative, eye catching campaigns that drive social media interactions as well as in office marketing materials. They have most certainly increased our social media presence while helping us transfer online interactions and referrals into paying, happy patients. Not only have they freed up our valuable staff from trying to manage our website, marketing and social media efforts, but they bring to the table a vast knowledge of industry market trends. They are a valued partner in our growing business."

-Chad A. Glazer, MD, Glazer Facial Plastic & Cosmetic Surgery, Michigan City, IN

"We loved how Kelly helped us streamline our event process. Helping us vet candidates, supplied excellent paperwork help, and really focused this experience for our patients in the most profitable way. She was simply the best!"

-Dr. McCormack, McCormack Plastic Surgery, Nevada

"This was so helpful! I learned so much about marketing and the phone scripts were so helpful. I was always too intimidated to call people and the (PGC) phone scripts don't sound salesy."

-Melinda Petersen, NuVista Plastic Surgery, Utah

"It was a very fun event, went just like clockwork. Event prep was well coordinated and made the evening run very smoothly. It was something that we will do again." SurgiCare Arts Aesthetics, Atlanta Georgia "We needed direction and planning help and it was 100% delivered! PGC helped with absolutely everything, she was attentive to all my requests and questions and did a wonderful job orchestrating the event with us. It was a major success! Thank you for helping us!"

-Dr. Coville, Cornerstone Plastic Surgery and Aesthetic Medicine, New Jersey

TOP 10 PROFIT KILLERS

FOR PLASTIC SURGEONS AND MEDICAL SPAS

And How to Avoid or Fix Them!

by

KELLY SMITH

Disclaimer

The material contained in this book is provided for educational and informational purposes only. The information provided is accurate and effective to the best of the author's knowledge. The author will not be held responsible for any outcome resulting from the use of this information.

ISBNs

978-1-7337436-4-8 *Hardback*

978-1-7337436-2-4 *Paperback*

978-1-7337436-3-1 *eBook*

Book design by Kelley Creative
www.kelleycreative.design

This book is dedicated to Chloe, Kole, and Karl, my loving family who are patient beyond measure! Thank you for allowing me the time to create a business that I love while making every effort to balance time and energy for you. My sister and parents have always been my biggest source of encouragement and strength and I am forever grateful to them for all the years of love and support.

As the leader of an all-female company and mother to a teenage girl, I want to celebrate women in business. The greatest joy I get in owning this company is from the amazing growth I see in the women on our team in both business and their personal lives. PGC is committed to creating opportunities for our team by consistently providing the opportunity for advancement, life balance, and positive impact for our clients and ourselves. I am grateful to have the opportunity to speak to groups of women in business and it is the highest compliment to be able to inspire and encourage women to dare to dream, set audacious goals, and share ideas for how to achieve them. ***In an effort to support and raise awareness of women's achievements we will donate a portion of the proceeds of this book to The Women's Entrepreneurship Day****, of which Projected Growth Consulting has been a long-term sponsor and an enthusiastic participant in their global and local events.*

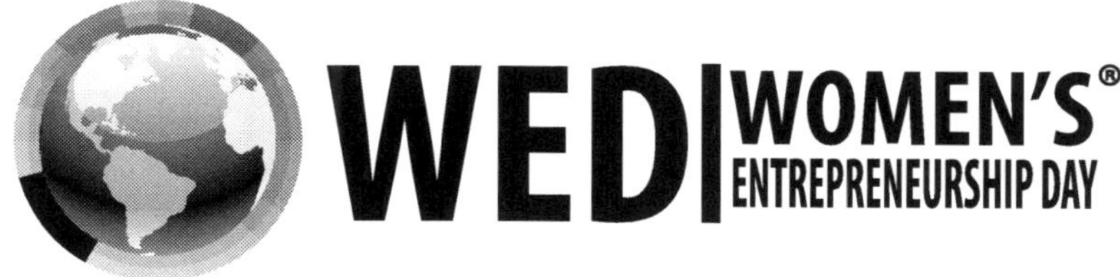

TABLE OF CONTENTS

INTRODUCTION

WHAT WE HAVE LEARNED FROM WORKING WITH THOUSANDS OF PRACTICES

After working with thousands of clinics, I created this book to let you see behind the scenes of elective medical practices to reveal the most common challenges. These are the top ten areas I have encountered that cause challenges for increasing revenue and profit. In the following, I will walk you through the top ten occurring mistakes and provide efficient and practical solutions to fix them or, better yet, avoid them altogether.

Even practices with a great bottom line may find one or more areas to focus on. Whether they are earning $1M or $5M, the challenges practices face are consistent, and they may have a few top priorities to work on. Every business suffers from at least two or more of these at any given time, although the areas of challenge may shift from year to year. You can use this book as a reference to solve challenges as priorities shift in your organization.

After running my own seven-figure medical spa in Eastern Washington, I was contracted by a laser and vein center in the Northwest to be their CFO on a turnaround project for two general surgeons. When I began to collaborate with them, the surgeons had been in business for eight years and reached their highest-ever sales per year of $800,000 with a marketing percentage of income exceeding 15%. The strategies in this book grew the revenue from $800,000 a year to over $4M a year in less than three years. As a result, the two general surgeons fulfilled their goal to become full-time cosmetic surgeons, which meant they could stop taking call rounds and insurance. On top of that, this growth enabled them to open a *second* location and to start two national training centers–all while reducing marketing expenses by 10%.

In 2009, soon after this success, I began speaking to and teaching physicians how to strategically handle their marketing and finance to create rapid profitability in their practices. Over the last decade, my consulting team has helped thousands of elective medical practices increase their profits, lower expenses, market more effectively, and create cohesive, top-selling teams.

My business consulting firm, Projected Growth Consulting (PGC), now helps an average of 40 practices a month nationally, and our results are consistent and replicable. I am writing this book to share some of the methods we use to create growth for our clients and their practices.

No matter the type of small business you own and operate or what industry you are in, three main areas of focus are finance, marketing, and operations. Each of these critical and commingled areas must be tended to by you or someone on your team.

The first step on your way to improvement involves a "physical" for your practice to assess how your business performs in ten key areas. To receive the most benefit from this exercise, take out a piece of paper and number it 1 to 10. On this list of ten items, you will utilize a scale from 1 to 10 to rate your practice's performance in each area outlined below.

You do not have to tell anyone else your answers, and your answers will not be graded like in medical school. However, you will receive the most from this book by taking an honest look at your situation. To fix a problem–just as you do with patients–we must first diagnose it. Systematic, proven ways exist to fix any problems you may have in your practice.

Keep in mind that nobody is a 10 in all areas. It is better to identify problem areas than to have all 10s and still not be profitable or able to reach your goals. Think of this self-assessment as your "before" snapshot, and imagine how delighted you will be to experience the "after."

The Projected Growth Consulting 10-Point Check-Up.

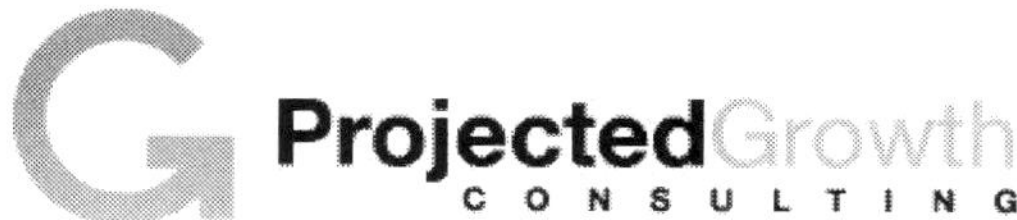

PGC 10-POINT CHECK-UP

	Answer Not Yet, Sometimes, or Yes.	Status
1	You have set monthly sales goals and measure performances weekly.	
2	You have written an Annual Marketing Plan and utilize it on a monthly basis.	
3	Your website is built for conversion, and you review analytic performances monthly	
4	You not only know your Practice Metrics and Industry Averages, but also measure them. These include industry averages for costs of goods, expenses, and pricing. You review your profit and loss monthly to track the costs and work to improve ratios.	
5	You have defined your Key Performance Indicators (KPIs) and marketing Return On Investment (ROI) and measure them monthly.	
6	You track lead conversions and consistently train staff to improve performance.	
7	You have a set consultation structure, track closing ratios, and close over 50%.	
8	You hold Sales Events, not open houses, on a quarterly basis.	
9	Social media is your lowest cost per lead, and you actively track results that produce growth consistently on your social media platforms, particularly Facebook and Instagram.	
10	You have created a positive company culture, and you and your team all enjoy going to work with each other!	
	PROVEN SYSTEMS CREATE PROVEN RESULTS!	

Keep a copy of your 10-point check-up. Revisit and rate these areas quarterly so you can see the incremental changes as they begin to happen. By measuring performance, you can acknowledge your progress and reward yourself and your team. Plus, studies show that the key to happiness is making measurable progress toward your goals.

We work with clients to solve these business challenges in one-hour strategy sessions. At first, an hour does not seem like much time. That is the point. Over the years, we observed many elective medical practices experiencing similar business challenges. And we became more efficient at pinpointing exactly which actions practices needed to take to improve. If you are like most of our clients, you are not seeking three more hours of meeting time in your already busy day. But any practice owner who desires positive change can dedicate an hour to strategic performance improvement in critical areas. Throughout my company's fifteen years of business consulting, we have continuously refined our processes and created proven systems, which produce predictable results for our clients.

My goal is to share these one-hour solutions with you, so you can grow your practice revenue and profit. Remember, I have been where you are. So this book outlines the common mistakes and how to fix them, in the order of importance and impact they have on your practice. Although these chapters are arranged in the order we use with clients, they can be prioritized based on your most critical areas of need. These proven systems exist to create success in elective medical practices, and you are about to learn and, hopefully, implement them. You can follow these chapters in order or begin with the areas most important to you.

Kelly Smith

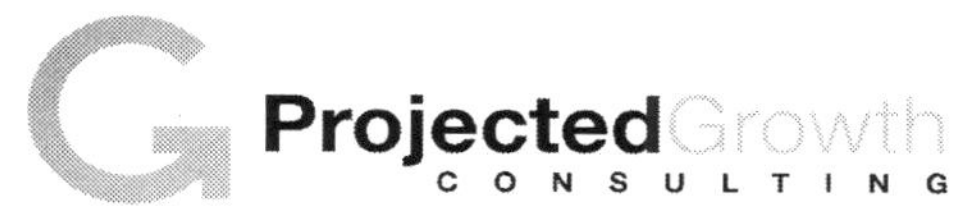

	BUSINESS ASSESSMENT - FINANCIAL	1= YES/ 0= NO
1	Do you know your average monthly sales?	
2	Do you measure revenue weekly?	
3	Do you have clear financial monthly goals?	
4	Do you have staff bonus structures?	
5	Do you review expenses quarterly?	
6	Do you have three or more key initiatives to increase net profit?	
7	Is your marketing percent of revenue between 5% and 15%?	
8	Is your labor cost of goods less than 25%?	
9	Is your net profit above 20%?	
10	Do you know your marketing ROI?	
	FINANCIAL SCORE	
	BUSINESS ASSESSMENT - OPERATIONS	1= YES/ 0= NO
1	Do you have written job descriptions for all staff?	
2	Do you do quarterly reviews?	
3	Do you hold regular weekly staff meetings?	
4	Do you have individual compensation plans for each staff member?	
5	Do you do monthly inventory and adjustments?	
6	Do you have more long-term employees than new employees?	
7	Do you provide staff free treatments?	
8	Do you pay retail commission?	
9	Does your staff know your mission or vision?	
10	Are you utilizing vendors to increase monthly profit?	
	OPERATIONAL SCORE	
	BUSINESS ASSESSMENT - MARKETING	1= YES/ 0= NO
1	Do you have a website?	
2	Is your site mobile enabled?	
3	Is your phone number on top of page, large, bold and clickable?	
4	Are your social media links on the top of page and do the links work?	
5	Have you been on your own site in the past month?	
6	Do you email clients specials regularly?	
7	Do you use Cross Promotions INSTEAD of Discounting?	
8	Do you respond to new leads within thirty minutes?	
9	Do you do a Gift Certificate of the Month on your homepage to get new leads?	
10	Is your Facebook following growing more than 20% per year?	
11	Do you do Facebook monthly giveaway contests?	
12	Do you have a goal with your social media posts? Share, comment?	
13	Do you have your own before and after photos on your website?	
14	Do you regularly post Vlogs or Blogs to your website and social media?	
15	Do you use Insights or other monthly analytics reports for online systems?	
16	Do you know your cost per lead?	
17	Do you know your practice closing ratio?	
18	Do you know how many consultations you need per month to hit your goals?	
19	Do you have an annual marketing plan?	
20	Do you do sales events instead of open houses?	
	TOTAL MARKETING SCORE	
	GRAND SCORE	

	BENCHMARKING - How are you doing?	SCORE
	WOW - YOU SHOULD TEACH THIS STUFF! CONGRATULATIONS!	30-40
	AVERAGE - WE CAN ROCK THIS PRETTY QUICKLY	20-29
	OUCH - WE NEED TO GIVE SOME ATTENTION ASAP	0-19

PROFIT KILLER #1

1. NO CLEAR AND MEASURABLE FINANCIAL PLAN

"Average revenues per facility are $924,000–with about 80% coming from procedures and 20% from retail product sales."[1]

Many of the clients we work with are at an average revenue of $800,000 to $1M. They come to us struggling with growth problems, and we are able to help them right away. They stall at about $800,000 and have trouble increasing to over $1M. It is our goal to get them into a more profitable revenue range. They seek our guidance or consulting to reach the next level. Once they reach that, their margins improve dramatically. Our typical client experiences a 30% growth in the first ninety days of our partnership.

If you feel uncomfortable with the financial analysis side of your business, you are not alone. The 1 Hour Revenue Plan, a strategic tool to set up your practice for financial success, can help you avoid failure. Knowledge is power. And the result of sharing clear sales goals while measuring performance builds collaboration and teamwork within your team.

Business owners tend to avoid looking at numbers or creating revenue projections because it can be overwhelming. When we break down the steps, the process becomes much more manageable.

Revenue Planning + Measuring Expenses = Financial Health

When it comes to the financial health of your practice, revenue and expenses are two main focus areas.

---

1 *Medical Spa Report: 3.6 billion US Market in 2016*, Medical Spa MD Blog

When you calculate revenue minus expenses, it equals net profit:

Revenue - Expenses = Net Profit

Your net profit amount is your taxable income.

In this chapter we focus solely on sales or revenue projections (one step at a time!) and how to measure them to create strategic growth in your practice. The goal is to set revenue projections to develop a profitable mix of services for your practice to create the highest net profit possible. Later we will look at margins, expenses, and industry averages.

First, review past sales results in order to set realistic sales projections. If possible, sort your revenue by category or service type so you can see the number of appointments and staff members and facility requirements necessary to produce your new sales goals. Begin by gathering key figures to start the process. I will identify the most important numbers to focus on through this chapter.

Monthly Revenue Worksheet and Weekly Status Report

The diagnostic tools you will need are the Monthly Revenue Worksheet and the Weekly Status Report in combination with a detailed profit and loss statement for at least the past twelve months or, preferably, longer. Previous performance numbers guide you in setting reasonable new sales thresholds.

If you are preparing to start a med spa or elective medical practice, begin with a conservative goal, such as growing by 20% per month. For now, let us assume you need ten appointments per week for the first month. The suggested growth per month will depend on your marketing budget, KPIs (Key Performance Indicators) and industry benchmarks, which I will explain in more detail in the following chapters.

If you have an existing practice, begin with your revenue to date this year and your monthly averages.

Divide your total sales or income by 12 to find out your average monthly revenue. If you are not sure, look at your monthly bank deposits and use those for your estimated total sales per month. Add together those estimated numbers and divide the total by the number of months included in your total sales to get your average. Optimally, as a starting benchmark, you should have two years or more to review by monthly sales, sales by service, and net profit percentages.

You can list services by the service name or treatment area. For example, you might use labels, such as toxins, fillers, photo facials, laser hair removal, face surgical, body surgical, breast surgical, hair transplantation, and retail. These categories can be broader, such as injectables, lasers, surgical, aesthetic services, and retail.

I suggest setting up your chart of accounts to match this tracking in order to have actionable intelligence for running your business. With narrower and more specific categories, it will be easier to make decisions based on profitability and vendor relationships.

If you are only tracking revenue or sales as one large number, now is an excellent time to divide it into the categories above. You can update or change your chart of accounts in your accounting software at month-end and make a note of when the new tracking begins. By tracking this way, you can see the direct costs of goods to these sales categories, which enables net profit analysis for increasing margins. That information will prove invaluable down the road. Below is a sample worksheet for guidance.

To download the two forms used in this chapter, visit the Resources Folder at the end of the book.

Sample Monthly Revenue Worksheet

ProjectedGrowth CONSULTING

REVENUE WORKSHEET

PRACTICE

DATE

Service	Last Year Total Revenue	Last Year Ave Mo Rev	Average Service Price	Services Per Month	Services Per Week	This Years Monthly Goals	Average Service Price	Services Per Month	Services Per Week
Body Surgical									
Face Surgical									
Other Surgical									
Vaginal Health									
Minimally Invasive Face									
Minimally Invasive Body									
Toxin									
Fillers									
Resurfacing									
IPL									
LHR									
Non Invasive Body									
Laser Misc									
Med Spa Aesthetics									
RX Skincare/Retail									
Other									
Other									
Other									
Total	$ -	$ -	$ -	0.00	0.00	$ -	$ -	0.00	0.00

Using the Worksheet

First, identify and list your own profit centers. Fill in the average monthly sales by service type. Next, calculate your monthly averages per service. Now, fill in your average sales price for each service type. Prices can have a broad range, so determine the average charge for the service.

If you offer laser hair removal, calculate an average price you charge per appointment–not the package price. For example, one laser hair removal session costs approximately $100. Now we can divide the average monthly revenue by the average cost per service to get an initial benchmark of the number of appointments you are currently doing on a monthly and weekly basis.

These benchmark numbers do not have to be exact right now. Depending on how you have set up your scheduling software, you may be able to print a sales report by profit center, as well as a report showing the average number of appointments per month by service type. If you can run these reports, do that now. If those reports are not available, doing this manually is a quick method to begin to understand how many appointments the practice has per month on average. If you track things well, you may be close to the real numbers. If not, at least you will be able to benchmark moving forward.

Our goal is to create a measurable process to see that appointments are increasing. The appointment analysis provides checks and balances for both staffing and capacity needs and necessary marketing budgets.

The service mix ratio is vital to the fiscal health of your practice. That is the ratio of revenue or percentage of sales coming from different profit centers. If you make 90% of your income from surgery, it can be challenging for the surgeon to enjoy time off without your practice experiencing steep income dips. Therefore, the goal is to have a healthy ratio or mix of surgical, ancillary, and retail services so your revenue can be predictable *and* allow for a vacation or a round of golf.

When assessing your profit centers, take time to review industry statistics. The ASPS (American Society of Plastic Surgeons) reported on cosmetic surgical procedures performed in 2018, and the top five were[2]:

1. Breast augmentation (313,735 procedures, up 4% from 2017)

2. Liposuction (258,558 procedures, up 5% from 2017)

3. Nose reshaping (213,780 procedures, down 2% from 2017)

4. Eyelid surgery (206,529 procedures, down 1% from 2017)

5. Tummy tuck (130,081 procedures, about the same as 2017)

These statistics[3] prove useful when considering how to diversify profit centers:

- Current non-invasive fat reduction and skin tightening procedures continue to gain popularity.

- Non-invasive fat reduction procedures that use special technology to freeze away fat without surgery increased by 7%.

- Non-surgical cellulite treatments that use lasers to eliminate fat increased by 19% (up 55% since 2000).

---

2 *New Plastic Surgery Statistics Reveal Trends Toward Body Enhancement*, plasticsurgery.org

3 New Statistics Reveal the Shape of Plastic Surgery, plasticsurgery.org

- Non-invasive skin tightening procedures that target fat and tighten sagging areas increased by 9%.

You might wonder how this works in the real world. A story about a client illustrates how revenue planning and ratios can enable you to work smarter—not harder.

How we helped a practice increase revenue by $1M within twelve months

Our client, a prominent and successful plastic surgeon with a 15-year-old practice, maintains a thriving business in Texas. After hiring our company to help them reach the next level, they hit a sales threshold of $3M. A single-surgeon practice, this doctor/owner deeply wanted to know how to produce income from other sources beyond surgery. However, it had proven extremely difficult to do. While the practice had good lasers, aesthetic services, and a retail variety, they were caught in a feast-or-famine cycle, and producing consistent sales in the med spa was a challenge.

As our first step we did what I showed you here. We analyzed revenue by service. Then we looked at the quantity of appointments and consultations. And finally, we reviewed surgical cases by category and size.

From that analysis we saw that we needed to increase retail sales to 10% of incoming revenue, triple laser and spa services, and adjust and plan the physician's surgical schedule and weekly case mix.

To ensure success, we:

- set goals for the staff on retail sales as a percentage of aesthetic services,

- modified the consultation format to include retail, ancillary, and surgical treatment plans,
- specified a template of how to book surgical cases weekly, and
- set up team sales goals and team bonuses for sales over targets.

The results were impressive.

The office compressed office hours from five and a half days a week to four and a half. They revised the surgical schedule to be set up for two body cases, four breast augmentation surgeries, and four shorter face- or miscellaneous cases a week. This new schedule meant the surgeon was in surgery three days a week and seeing patients in consultations and follow-ups on the fourth day. Then there was a half-day for administrative and other follow-up tasks as needed. This half-day was only twice per month.

Schedule delays decreased and patient complaints decreased. By segregating surgery from consultations and follow-up appointments, the day ran on time. Patient and staff complaints were reduced, and the physician's stress levels went down!

They became booked six weeks in advance. The plan enabled staff to confidently schedule surgeries further into the future, instead of acting on the impulse to squeeze them in as soon as possible. Soon they were booked out six weeks in advance. The result took the overload off the staff and the surgeon, and also created consistent monthly revenue.

The staff received regular bonuses tied to performance. The practice implemented retail sales commissions and etiquette to recommend one to three products at the close of every checkout. Clear revenue goals were set for the next twelve months and communicated to the staff. They saw the group sales performance numbers each week. If they made it over the goal, then everyone received a team bonus.

For every $10,000 the office finished over the goal, each team member received $100. Before long, they got used to $400-per-month bonuses. They added quarterly Sales Events and stopped discounting. They implemented monthly cross-promotions to combine injectables or lasers with surgery cases to increase revenue for those ancillary non-surgical services.

Small changes over time can create significant results.

Within twelve months, the office was up $1M in sales, *and* they were working one day less per week. That year, the doctor took the team on a Caribbean cruise as a reward.

The key lessons from this case study are:

- create clear sales goals by profit center,
- measure sales performances weekly and reward the staff as a team,
- add retail commission and a protocol to meet the client at checkout to talk about the products to help build the retail numbers.

Understanding how many and what type of cases they needed for surgery, they began to create a predictable income and avoid significant fluctuations. The staff makes more money working one day less, and the physician now has 40% of the income mix of the practice coming from non-surgical services. Now he can even take a vacation, and the practice will still generate revenue from the ancillary non-surgical services.

In the next chapter, we will cover how to cross-promote and create your Annual Marketing Plan to build these kinds of results. However, it all starts with a thorough analysis of where the revenue currently comes from. When you know this, you can create the best cross-promotions and event schedules to increase the services that will benefit your practice the most.

To encourage teamwork, you must set clear sales goals for the month and measure sales performances weekly. These two steps will create excitement, teamwork, and motivation for the practice. Rewarding your staff as a team creates a good company culture and minimizes the amount of time spent on staff management and oversight. The "What's in it for me?" factor applies as much to internal staff as it does to your external customers.

Below is the weekly status report that we use to motivate the team. This tool takes only minutes per week to maintain. If tools require too much time and effort to use, we simply do not use them. That is why I created this simple Weekly Revenue Calculator, which you can download in the Resources Folder at the end of the book (PDF or working Excel version).

Weekly Revenue Tracker

Reporting Ending Date:	
For the Month of:	
Fill in Yellow at Month Start	
Fill in Green Each Monday	
Current Month to Date Revenue	$ 25,000.00
Monthly Revenue Goals	$ 40,000.00
$ Variance	$ 15,000.00
% of Plan Completed	63%
Number of Working Days in Month	20
Number of Days Worked So Far	11
Number of Days Left in Month	9
% Month Completed	55%
% Variance	8%
Daily Revenue Average	$ 2,272.73
Daily Revenue Goal Now	$ 1,666.67
Forecasted Month	$ 45,454.55
% Projected Goal	114%

Bonus Calculator

Monthly Breakeven	$ 40,000.00
This Month Revenue Projected	$ 45,454.55
Performance Over Plan	$ 5,454.55
Bonus 1%	$ 54.55

This system's color coding makes it simple to use. Enter your sales revenue goal on the first of the month and the number of days your practice will see patients this month. Then enter the total sales goal for the week before you open on Monday morning and update the number of days worked so far that month. After that, print out the results and post them in the breakroom for your team to view. This critical step allows the team to modify behavior and strategies to make the goal. If it makes you nervous to share these numbers, consider how you can expect the staff to meet or exceed your sales goals if they do not know what they are. That is like jumping into your car and being mad at the navigation system when you do not arrive at your desired destination, even though you never entered it into the system in the first place.

When you set monthly sales goals, you need to share the previous years of sales and then increase them by 10% or more if you have new technology or staff, or if your marketing brings in additional clients. You can raise the goals dramatically if you show the team the number of weekly appointments it will take to get there by treatment type and what you are doing in the business to make that possible. For example, you might have purchased a new microneedling pen and HydraFacial machine, hired extra staff to increase capacity, or increased your online marketing budget to attract additional new patients.

Measured performance *improves.* The concept of open-book accounting may feel uncomfortable for some physicians or practice managers. Part of educating your staff about business involves explaining the difference between revenue or sales and net profit. Look at it this way: Informed employees are not as quick to go out and open an injectable business on their own once they understand the reality of what it costs to provide the services.

This basic business knowledge will prove helpful when negotiating compensation plans with your staff members. An employee needs to generate four times their cost to the organization to make sense of the hire, which we will discuss in detail later. Talking about net profit versus sales helps in this discussion and also in the compensation negotiation. You get less push back with clear sales goals and benchmarks. For example, once you teach them that 20% net profit is a healthy bottom line, then you can walk them through what it costs to own and operate a practice. Explaining these concepts with real numbers is critical. Since many people's eyes often glaze over when numbers are discussed, it is important to meet them at their level and speak in basic language. The following exemplifies how to communicate this baseline knowledge to your team:

Every $1,000 that comes in from sales, which is our income or revenue, translates into only $200 or 20% of net profit. In other words, after rent, payroll, marketing, costs of goods to render services, utilities, taxes, and professional fees required to run the practice, the reality is that only 20%, or $200, is what you actually earn for every $1,000 of income. So, for $1M of sales, the profit will be $200,000.

Let us say you have an RN doing injectables at your practice, and she thinks she could earn more doing it on her own. Would it not be helpful for her to have a realistic idea of what that would really mean to her in terms of income? Over the years this conversation with the supporting numerical breakdown has stopped many talented, large-volume injectable nurses from leaving our clients' thriving practices.

Let us say the RN is injecting $50,000 a month–$600,000 a year–in toxins and filler revenue or sales for the practice. Since the cost of goods or injectable product cost is 50% on average, this leaves a $300,000 profit for the year once we subtract the costs of products. If her income is $100,000 annually, we are left with a $200,000 profit for the year.

If she entered into business on her own, the numbers tell a much worse story of the money she will earn for the time and money spent. Let us say she gets a deal on rent for only $3,000 per month and hires only one staff member in the form of a front desk receptionist (assistant/inventory manager/office cleaner all in one!) for another $3,000 a month. Those two costs bring the annual profit down by $72,000, leaving only $128,000 per year. That translates into a monthly profit of less than $11,000.

That still sounds good. However, we have not yet subtracted marketing costs, phone, power, taxes, accounting fees, laundry, and all other expenses. To generate $50,000 in monthly sales, you need a marketing budget of 5% at the lowest, or $2,500 per month, for a total of $30,000 per year. If we then add taxes and a small accounting budget, we arrive at $666.67 per month extra income plus all of the responsibilities and liabilities of owning the business.

Injectable Income/Year	$600,000.00
Cost of Product/Year	$300,000.00
Profit/Year	$300,000.00
Injector Wages/Year	$100,000.00
Profit/Year	$200,000.00
Rent/Year	$36,000.00
Staffing/Year	$36,000.00
Profit/Year	$128,000.00
Profit/Month	10,666.67
5% Marketing/Year	$30,000.00
5% Marketing/Month	$2,500.00
Monthly Profit	$8,166.67
Accounting/Month	$250.00
Taxes Annual Taxes	$90,000.00
Monthly Taxes	$7,500.00
Monthly Profit Remaining	$666.67

The full numbers tell the full story. She has a better deal staying at the practice instead of opening a location on her own. But without any framework or education about profitability versus sales, she might assume she would make more money on her own. Hopefully, this helps you see the benefit in educating your staff rather than keeping them in the dark. You reap cost savings by keeping staff. That way you do not have to spend more on recruiting and hiring or potentially lose patients, who may follow a provider who leaves.

Understanding numbers to avoid over-compensation

If you do not understand your numbers and ratios, you might make the common mistake of offering a staff member a revenue split–say, something like a 30% split of injectable sales or laser treatments. Owners often strike these deals in the beginning of their practices to save money, because they do not want to pay staff if they do not have enough appointments to keep them busy. The thought of paying an hourly rate or salary if the staff member is not busy seems like a waste of money. This is a tough problem to solve, as cutting a compensation plan typically ends with your employee leaving, and not happily. Unfortunately, I encounter several practices every year where this shortsighted error has been made. As shown in the Revenue Tracker above, if you agreed to a 30% split in that same scenario, you would be losing money on injectable revenue, a very critical area of your business. These numbers are vital to your success and business profitability.

An educated staff is your best staff. Set realistic sales goals by service and adjust for seasonality and events. Then post the goals for the year for your staff to see. Do not change the sales goal once the month begins. That is not fair. I suggest adjusting quarterly at the most. Take your time to set the goals carefully and then reward the team for working together to achieve them. Show them the results weekly so they have time to correct or work together to increase sales.

Suddenly you will find your staff doing follow-up calls without being nagged. They may meet with a vendor and get a deal on a product or do a phone campaign to pre-sell injectables. I have seen amazing results from this one practice management tool. What do you have to lose? You will only pay bonuses above achieved goals, which is above breakeven. If you have ten employees, you are giving up 10% of the sales revenue as a bonus of the sales you probably would not have had without this incentive. The other 90% is the profit in the business minus your expenses. I have seen firsthand how this proven method has dramatically changed hundreds of practices for the better.

Complete the 1 Hour Revenue Plan now and you will be well on your way to completing the recommendations in this chapter and making your business grow.

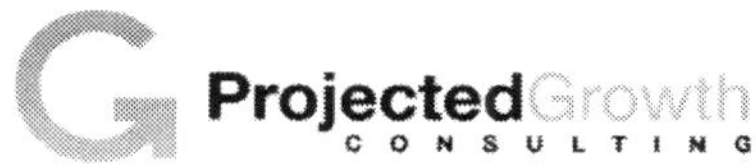

1 HOUR REVENUE PLAN

	Action Items to Complete	Who	Due Date	Status
1	Run sales reports from your CRM to see what is available			
2	Download the Monthly Revenue Worksheet			
3	Download the Weekly Revenue Tracker			
4	Print your profit and loss statements for the past 3 years			
5	Document your annual revenue for past 3 years			
6	Calculate your average monthly revenue for each year of data			
7	List your profit centers and services			
8	Run a revenue report for the past 12 months			
9	Calculate your averge monthly sales for the past 12 months			
10	Enter your average price per service			
11	Calculate services per month averages past 12 months			
12	Calculate services per week averages past 12 months			
13	Set revenue goals by service - 10% over last year for the same month			
14	Calculate monthly appointments to meet new goals			
15	Calculate weekly appointments to meet new goals			
16	Fill in the monthly revenue sheet			
17	Fill in the revenue tracker with sales goals			
18	Edit your Chart of Accounts to match new profit center list			
19	Review that staffing and capacity can handle new goals			
20	Implement Revenue Tracker			
21	Review sales weekly			
22	Set day of the week for status reports to be due			
23	Create Employee Team Bonus Plan			
24	Implement Team Bonus with start date			
25	Set up team meeting to explain the process			
	PROVEN SYSTEMS CREATE PROVEN RESULTS!			

PROFIT KILLER #2

2. LACK OF AN ANNUAL MARKETING PLAN (AMP)

Working with more than 1,000 physicians in the aesthetics industry over the past decade, we have seen that the three key areas of strategy required for growth and profit are *finance*, *operations*, and *marketing*. Of all the systems and processes that can help your practice take revenue and profit to the next level, the most impactful strategy to market and grow your practice is to implement an Annual Marketing Plan (AMP).

A solid AMP helps you increase revenue, decrease impulsive marketing spending, direct patients into new services, maintain your bottom line, smooth out cash flow, and create high surges of revenue through quarterly Sales Events. Without the AMP in place, the result is often stagnation, confusion, and the need to discount.

The four key essentials of an AMP are:

1. Monthly cross-promotions
2. Social media planning
3. E-mail marketing
4. Quarterly Sales Events

Implementing an AMP increases profitability and organization and yields happy patients and repeat business. By strategically narrowing your marketing focus and strengthening the cohesion and layering of your overall message, you will reach new clients and increase conversion and closing ratios of existing and new patients.

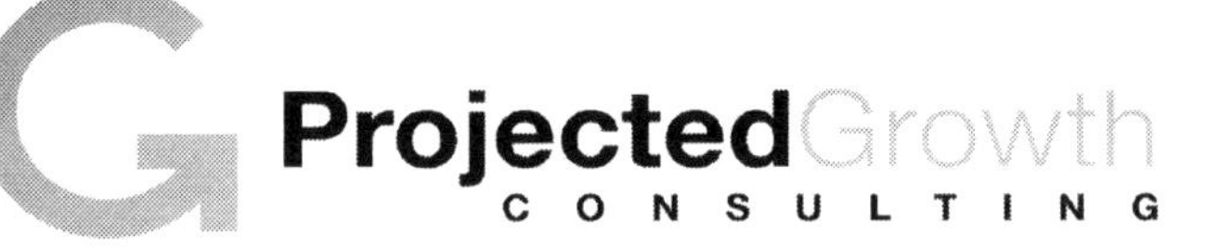

ProjectedGrowth
CONSULTING

	MARKETING DIAGNOSTIC ANALYSIS	YES =1/ NO =0
1	Do you know your top three competitors?	
2	Do you track your conversion ratio from lead to consult?	
3	Do you track your current average closing ratio per month?	
4	Do you know your average practice income?	
5	Do you have a monthly revenue goals?	
6	Do you measure your revenue weekly?	
7	Do you have a client e-mail List?	
8	Do you update that list monthly?	
9	Do you know your average cost per lead?	
10	Do you email your clients weekly with different content and offers?	
11	Do you have formalized incentives for staff to up sell or cross sell?	
12	Do you pay retail commission to staff?	
13	Do you do cross promotions and avoid straight discounting?	
14	Do you track the lead source in your system for all new clients?	
15	Do you run a report quarterly to look at which lead sources are the best?	
16	Do you look at your marketing budget by line item quarterly?	
17	Are you currently getting at least a 400% ROI on your marketing dollars spent?	
18	Do you spend 5-10% of revenue on marketing?	
19	Do you have an SEO program?	
20	Are you consistently doing a PPC campaign?	
21	Do you utilize sales funnel methods to follow and drip on your leads?	
22	Do you have paid advertising on your FB or Instagram?	
23	Do you know the top ten selling skin care products you sell?	
24	Do you sell 10% or more of your revenue in RX Skin Care?	
25	Do you automatically send out e-mails requesting patient reviews?	

26	Is your confirmation process automated by email or texting?	
27	Do you have an automated way to post good reviews on line?	
28	Do you utilize COME back discounts or gift cards?	
29	Do you do quarterly event for patients to have the opportunity to save money?	
30	Do you offer discounts at any other time than events?	
31	Do you offer Botox Party programs?	
32	Do you have a client appreciation or VIP event each year?	
33	Do you have an annual marketing plan by month for the year?	
34	Do you offer a referral reward to current patients for referring friends?	
35	Can all of your staff members answer questions about all of your services?	
36	Can all of your staff answer general pricing questions for your services?	
37	Do you have a loyalty points program for your clients?	
38	Do you have a consistent system to reactivate former patients?	
39	Do you have a process or system to follow up on closed consultations?	
40	Do you have your email list segmented by patient types and targets?	
41	Is the average number of patient referrals increasing?	
42	Do you write articles or blogs and post on your website monthly?	
43	Do you do regular video and post on social platforms and website monthly?	
44	Do you have a YouTube channel?	
45	Do you regularly use Facebook?	
46	Is your Facebook following increasing by over 20% per year?	
47	Do you post on Facebook 4-7 times per week?	
48	Do your social links work on mobile and your website?	
49	Do you post on Instagram 4-7 times per week?	
50	Do you run a monthly contest on Facebook and Instagram for products or services?	
	Totals	

	BENCHMARKING - How are your doing?	**YES =1/ NO =0**
	WOW - YOU SHOULD TEACH THIS STUFF! CONGRATULATIONS	OVER 25
	AVERAGE - WE CAN ROCK THIS PRETTY QUICKLY	11 TO 24
	OUCH - WE NEED TO GIVE SOME ATTENTION ASAP	UNDER 10

Case Study: Doubling Net Profit in Thirteen Months While Decreasing Marketing Budget by 15%

A practice-based med spa in Louisiana came to us because their marketing costs negatively impacted profitability. After seven years in business, the team struggled to create growth without spending all of their profits on lead generation and marketing.

We recommended an AMP that shifted the focus of their marketing efforts by replacing their discounting strategy with cross-promotions, implementing monthly social media contests, and e-mailing their existing client database on a weekly basis.

As a result, they experienced a dramatic increase in sales for their most profitable service–a minimally invasive procedure. Within thirteen months they doubled their net profit *despite decreasing their marketing spending by 15%*. By implementing these three key marketing efforts, they continue to experience patient loyalty and referrals.

Case Study: 30% Increase in Elective Profits Within Six Months

A thriving California-based dermatology practice team found it challenging to incorporate elective aesthetics despite being well published and highly respected in the industry.

We helped them implement an AMP to create monthly cross-promotions focused on new elective aesthetics. We recommended introducing a weekly marketing e-mail and social media campaign directed to their existing client base to increase awareness of new injectable and laser services.

Within six months, elective profits increased by 30%. The practice experienced so much growth that they needed to hire an additional PA solely to focus on the elective profit center.

Targeting Your Ideal Client

In the aesthetics industry women between the ages of 19 and 64 comprise the majority of your target clientele. Men typically constitute about 10% of a practice's patient base. As you are designing your AMP, consider where and how you find your patients. Your most important lead sources include online, patient and staff referrals, and your current patient base. I will show you how to target these sources with every element of your marketing plan, so you will receive the maximum benefit.

Studies have shown that people need to see a message eight to ten times before they will respond to it.[4] A decade ago, this would have been three to five times, and the figure continues to grow as we are exposed to an increasing amount of input with each passing minute. Our phones ping us with e-mails. We hear commercials on the radio and see them on television, in print, and online. As a marketer or advertiser, you need to layer your messaging to capture the attention of your audience and sell to people when they are ready to buy.

Key Elements of an AMP

Cross-promotions give clients what they want for free as a reward for trying something new. This method works exceptionally well in the aesthetics industry in terms of creating exposure for a product or service that might be difficult to sell on its own. Let us say your cross-promotion offers a free toxin with a laser series–you automatically have two talking points for the month. Toxins, series, and medical grade retail products are particularly suitable for cross-promotion because they are typically done quarterly.

Facebook/Instagram monthly giveaway contests yield the best social media marketing results for our clients. A contest provides the WIIFM (*What's in it for me?*) that engages followers, so they will comment, like, and share your offers. Having managed social media for years, we have seen this tactic alone triple the growth

4 *Rule of 7: How Social Media Crushes Old-School Marketing,* Kruse Control Inc.

for our clients. Comments and shares are direct recommendations from your followers to their friends and associates. The primary goal of social media marketing is to create online referrals that become a lead source.

E-mail marketing is a fantastic means of communicating with an audience who has signed up to receive information from your practice. When a client gives you their personal e-mail, it is a token of trust. That is why it is imperative that every e-mail you send offers value for them. We have found that sending a weekly e-mail to your patient database yields the highest response. A variety of topics can be used to interest your patients in the other services you offer.

Quarterly Sales Events are another key element in your AMP. These have proven extremely effective for conversion. Keep a narrow focus for each event: body, breasts, face, feminine health, body contouring, or injectables. Pre-qualifying attendees is the best way to ensure high conversion at events. The event is not an open house; it is a consultation in the round. You can incentivize attendance by awarding door prizes and a grand prize at the event. Limit event capacity to thirty attendees to allow enough time for each interested patient to spend fifteen minutes in private consultation with the physician.

How to Build Your AMP

- **What:** Create an entire year's marketing plan in one hour. The key elements of the AMP are monthly cross-promotions, Sales Events, and social media content.

- **Why:** Our goal is to attract new clients and sell deeper to our existing client base. I will explain what makes this unique in the aesthetics industry.

- **How:** Using a Gantt chart as our AMP tool, I will teach you how to fill in your monthly marketing plan.

The Gantt chart below shows a sample AMP divided into monthly segments. For each month, we have highlighted the relevant focus area for cross-promotions, social media giveaway contests, blog and vlog topics, quarterly Sales Events, and website maintenance tasks. I will walk you through how to prepare your own chart.

#	Sample Annual Marketing Plan	J	F	M	A	M	J	J	A	S	O	N	D	Campaign	Offer or Date	Savings
1	Monthly Specials - This Mo On	J	F	M	A	M	J	J	A	S	O	N	D	Post on website, FB, In office, E-blast each Tuesday.	Limited to…people	Value of offer?
1.1	10 Years Younger This Year													Free Botox with Clear & Brilliant Series	5	$ 200.00
1.2	Lips and Lashes for Cupid													Free Latisse with any filler	5	$ 160.00
1.3	Shed your spots for spring													Free Microderm with IPL Series	10	$ 300.00
2	FaceBook Monthly Contest	J	F	M	A	M	J	J	A	S	O	N	D	Post 1st, award month end	Varied Prizes	Value of offer?
2.1	Botox													Free Botox 20 unites		$ 200.00
2.2	Filler													Free Latisse with any filler		$ 160.00
2.3	IPL													Free IPL		$ 300.00
3	2 Blogs/2 Vlogs Per Mont	J	F	M	A	M	J	J	A	S	O	N	D	You Tube, Webstie, Blog, Social Media	Week 1 & 3	Week 2 & 4
3.1	10 Years Younger This Year													Free Botox with Clear & Brilliant Series	Toxin	Clear & Brilliant
3.2	Lips and Lashes for Cupid													Free Latisse with any filler	Latisse	Filler
3.3	Shed your spots for spring													Free Microderm with IPL Series	IPL	Microderm
4	Quarterly On Site Events	J	F	M	A	M	J	J	A	S	O	N	D	Concept and Prizes	RSVP's	Sales Goal
4.1	New Year New You													Body Event, 20% Savings, Grand Prize	30	Goal $50,000
4.2	Look 10 Years Younger													Injectable, Lasers, Retail, 20% off, Grand Prize	30	Goal $30,000
4.4	Exclusive VIP Event													Swag Bag, Discount Packages, Invite Only	30	Goal $40,000
5	Website Maintenance	J	F	M	A	M	J	J	A	S	O	N	D	Ongoing Website Tasks	Due Date	By Whom
5.1	Event Calendar													Update content, winners and blogs and photos	Quarterly	Office Manager
5.2	Monthly Specials													Post all in January for the year or quarterly	Quarterly	Office Manager

Examine your current marketing efforts using the Marketing Self Diagnostic Assessment located in the Diagnostic Tools section of the Resources Chapter at the end of this book. Identify the areas in which you wish to improve performance. Next, take a few minutes to fill in the self-survey to identify the strategies that may be missing from your current marketing plan.

You may find it useful to revisit both of these tools on a quarterly basis as a benchmarking tool to track progress.

Using Your AMP

To make the marketing plan do-able, we break it down into quarterly, monthly, weekly, and daily tasks that you can schedule in your calendar.

- Quarterly tasks: Update website, promote events

- Monthly tasks: Cross-promotion, Facebook giveaway contest, update social media cover art

- Weekly tasks: Post on social media four to seven times, post blog, post vlog, e-mail client list, post vlog on website

- Daily tasks: Respond to comments on social media

Cross-Promotions

We all know how hard it is to resist the offer of a free gift with purchase. As customers, we want the free Lancôme bag with the lipsticks that are not really our color, so we will buy the eye shadow palette and the mascara. We have helped our clients sell millions of dollars' worth of aesthetics and med spa services, procedures, and products. Through this work, we have learned what it takes to win sales in this tough industry, and cross-promotions are the key to selling more.

While deep discounting can work for some practices, most cannot afford to consistently offer them. Although discounts of 50% will bring in a few people, that does not necessarily mean you are selling more. Offering clients what they want for free as a reward for trying something new provides an effective method for bringing exposure to something that is difficult for you to sell on its own. BOTOX® and fillers are fantastic for cross-promotions. For example, you could cross-promote BOTOX® or Dysport® with microneedling, microdermabrasion or dermaplaning. In a cross-promotion, the service you offer for free should be something you know your clients love. This keeps your clients coming back every six or eight weeks.

Speaking of having your clients regularly return to your practice, we encourage our clients to focus on programs that encourage patients to come back. BOTOX® parties, loyalty programs, VIP events, and referral reward systems are a key part of growing your existing client base and increasing net practice profit. As it turns out, "*Loyal customers that purchase from you frequently are much more profitable than your average customer, [and] your loyal top 10% spend 3x more per order than the lower 90%, and your top 1% of customers spend 5x more than the lower 99%.*"[5]

With cross-promotions, the value added should amount to a discount of *at least 20%* to ensure success. Offering less than this will likely prove ineffective. With surgery, you will want to add injectables as the added value. With new lasers, you can cross-promote with retail medical-grade products or ancillary services such as microneedling or microdermabrasion.

When selecting which two of your services or products to cross-promote, consider the following factors:

- Seasonality
- Potential cost and profit

5 *29 Ecommerce Metrics & KPIs to Measure to Drive 10X Growth in 2019*, Big Commerce as quoted in *Repeat Customers Are Profitable And We Can Prove It*, Smile.io

- Which new treatments or services you would like to introduce or promote
- Your current clientele's favorite treatments or services
- Vendor assistance with free products or treatments

Which of the following are you trying to be? Check three descriptors that apply to your practice.

☐	Clinical atmosphere	☐	Med spa atmosphere
☐	Luxury (cosmetic/ plastic surgery) atmosphere	☐	Brand built on physician expertise and reputation
☐	Emphasis on retail products	☐	Emphasis on procedures
☐	A few elective aesthetic services	☐	Non-invasive to minimally invasive treatments
☐	Full range of treatments and services		

- Which services do you want to grow?
- Which areas are most profitable?
- Which are your favorite services to offer?
- What is your main challenge?

The answers to these questions will tell you which procedures, treatments, and products to use for cross-promotions.

Remember to take seasonality into consideration when selecting monthly cross-promotions and scheduling quarterly events. This encourages a net profit-focused strategy for your AMP.

The two services you focus on in your cross-promotion should drive the whole marketing plan for that month. Layer your monthly cross-promotion messaging by featuring it on your website, spreading it across all your social media platforms, highlighting it in your e-mails, and displaying it on flyers in your office. This ensures that no matter how or where people hear from you, your message remains consistent.

Consistency of messaging boosts search engine optimization (SEO). A website optimized for search engines will appear more often when your prospective customers search online for what you offer. Our goal is to get people to phone us, to engage with our social media platforms, and to reach out to us via the contact form on our website–all of these constitute leads. Selling deeper to our existing patient base and attracting new clients result in more people walking through our door, which ultimately creates increased revenue.

Promotion Graphics

When you have selected your cross-promotions for the entire year–one per month for twelve months–it is time to create twelve promotion graphics to help you advertise them. As you build a graphic for your cross-promotion, keep in mind that more than 70% of your web views will be on a mobile device–and probably while the viewer is on the move and quickly scanning information. This means that you will want to use very few words.

Your promotion graphic should contain the following elements:

- Headline
- Offer

- Three or four main benefits or expected results

- Offer value

- Call to action (CTA): e.g. *click to book, call for a consultation,* or *click here to accept this offer*

Your headline needs to hook the reader and compel them to read further. Directly below it, you should mention the *value added*—essentially the two procedures or services you are cross-promoting.

Make sure to include three or four benefits of each procedure (or of its expected results).

The call to action compels the viewer to act on the offer by clicking the link or picking up the phone. It is best to appeal to their emotions while emphasizing urgency:

- *While supplies last!*

- *This month only!*

- *First 5 patients!*

Look at the graphics below and consider how they achieve each of the elements we have just discussed.

Chin up
THIS SUMMER
Limited to first 5
FREE DYSPORT with
Purchase of KYBELLA
($500 value)
Benefits of Kybella
• Contours & Reduces Fat Under the Chin
• Non-Surgical, Non-Invasive, No Downtime
• 15 Minute In-Office Appointment

Image: Select an image that really supports the idea you are trying to communicate. The image should be striking to grab the viewer's attention while having the emotional impact mentioned earlier.

In this busy marketplace, attention is practically your future revenue. Every practice will have its own style. It is essential to carefully consider what type of image will appeal to the demographic in your area. Some markets may lean more conservative (for example Lincoln, Nebraska). Other markets might be more liberal in their tastes and respond well to more flashy or edgy images (perhaps Miami, Florida).

You can visit www.shutterstock.com and www.stock.adobe.com to source stock images to use on your promotion graphic without infringing copyrights.

After you have created your promotion graphic, be sure to save your document both in JPG and PDF formats.

EVERYTHING IS
BRIGHTER IN
THE SUMMER!
FREE BOTOX®
with Purchase
of IPL Series
($260 Value)

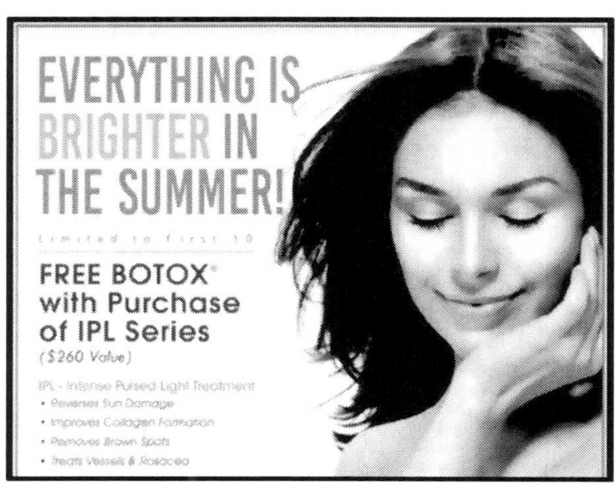

Print version (PDF): The PDF is for printing. Make sure your printed flyer is scattered around the practice where people can see it. Display a large flyer in a pretty frame at the front desk, and position stacks of takeaway flyers in the waiting room, treatment rooms, and restrooms for patients to take home. This will inspire patients to initiate conversations with your staff and build awareness of your promotion and of the services you provide.

Online version (JPG): The JPG is for sharing online. Upload it to your website and share it via Facebook, Instagram, and other social media platforms you are using, as well as in your e-mail marketing.

Action Items to Complete	Who	Date
Research a few stock photo sites		
Create a stock photo site account		
Purchase a stock photo plan on the site for buying images		
Start saving images for your promotion graphics		
Determine who will be responsible for creating the promotion graphics (in-house staff or outside marketer)		
Complete your first quarter of promotion graphics (3)		
Post on website, Facebook, Instagram		

Social Media Integration and Giveaway Contests

Results of a study published in the December 2018 issue of the *Aesthetic Surgery Journal* showed that patients base their choice of plastic surgeon more on their practice's Google rating and social media presence than on the surgeon's education and experience.[6] We have long suspected this, and this report confirms it based on unbiased research.

The article states, "Having a strong social media is what now drives patients to plastic surgeons' offices." The release continues, "Patients have increasingly been using online resources to make healthcare decisions and have a tendency to trust and value the rating that providers receive online."

Below are some notable statistics from "The Ultimate List of Marketing Statistics for 2018" (posted on HubSpot)[7].

- 79% of people online use Facebook.
- 76% of adults use Facebook daily.
- As of June 2018, Facebook had 1.47 billion daily active users.
- Instagram hit 1 billion monthly users in June 2018.
- As of January 2018, the age group with the most Instagram users worldwide is 18-24, followed by 25-34.
- Millennials check their phones over 150 times a day.
- Americans spend 5 hours per day on their mobile devices.

You may be thinking, *"Is social media really that important?"* There is no doubt your clients view social media. Digital marketing has replaced most traditional marketing methods. Let us look at some social media statistics before we get into the details of

6 *Aesthetic Surgery Journal*, December 2018.
7 *The Ultimate List of Marketing Statistics for 2018*, HubSpot

how content, consistency, and contests achieve your lowest cost per lead. We all know that patient, physician, or staff referrals are the highest converting lead source. Social media is nothing more than a warm referral–friend to friend. The right social media will make your followers smile, fall in love with your practice and your staff, and feel like an insider!

Social media and video-viewing are the two most popular online activities.

- 100 million hours of video content are watched daily on Facebook.[8]
- 64% of users are more likely to buy a product online after watching a video.[9]

You can create brand awareness, reach, impressions, and action by using social media to connect with both your current clients and potential clients in your demographic. Engagement is key. In order to increase revenue via your social platforms, you must engage your followers.

Hands down, the best results we have achieved on social media come from monthly giveaway contests on Facebook. We have managed social media on a monthly basis for dozens of clients, and the giveaway contest is a surefire method for keeping followers engaged. Engaged followers will likely share your content, and that is when you experience exponential growth.

Outline your monthly contests for twelve months in your AMP. Switching up the format of your giveaway contest periodically reinvigorates any slipping engagement and provides variety for your hard-core followers. For example, you can do a surprise giveaway prize or run a You Vote contest and let your followers choose from three options. When applicable, we recommend that you connect the prize to the monthly cross-promotion. If you are

8 *Facebook Hits 100M Hours of Content Watched a Day, 1B Users on Groups, 80M on Fb Lite*, TechCrunch.com.

9 *Video Marketing: The Future of Content Marketing*, Forbes.com.

offering a free series of chemical peels with a facial procedure, you might also offer a chemical peel as the giveaway prize for the month-long contest on Facebook and Instagram. Later in this book, I will go into more detail about how to run a social media contest.

Ask yourself the following questions:

1. Who in our practice is responsible for posting to social media?
2. Do we have the log-ins to all our social media platforms?
3. Do we have Facebook and Instagram profiles? Are these set up as business Pages?
4. Do we have a social media manager?

E-mail Marketing

Share news of events, flash sales, monthly promotions, and special offers from your vendors by e-mail. Vary the format so you are not sending the same type of content each week.

Subject line: Your e-mail subject line is critical to the deliverability of your campaign. Studies have shown that 33% of people open an e-mail based on whether or not they like the subject line, and 69% of people will report an e-mail as spam based on the subject line alone.[10] Here are a few tips for developing a great subject line in the aesthetics industry:

- **Pique the reader's curiosity.** Give them a brief idea about what is in the e-mail but keep it mysterious enough that they cannot resist opening it to read the rest.

10 *22 Eye-Opening Statistics About Sales E-mail Subject Lines That Affect Open Rates,* HubSpot.

- **Add urgency, but only when the offer is time-sensitive.** If you are trying to collect RSVPs for an upcoming event, feel free to infuse the subject line with a sense of urgency. However, it must really be time-sensitive. If the e-mail is not time-sensitive, the reader may feel disgruntled that you have tricked them into opening it, and that can result in a higher unsubscribe rate.

- **Keep it short and sweet.** As most readers are viewing on their mobile devices, shorter subject lines are better. You would not want them to miss the most important piece of the subject line.

Content: Marketing e-mails do not always have to contain a promotional offer. E-mails are a great way to share links to your blog posts, announce giveaways, and send holiday greetings. When sharing content, always include a title, an image, and a short excerpt of the text, and link to the original post on your blog.

Images: Most e-mail servers cannot handle a large image. It is best to keep images between 600 and 800 pixels wide.

Scheduling: Your AMP should include weekly e-mails to your patient database. Studies show that e-mailing clients once a week yields the highest response.[11] In the aesthetics industry, we recommend weekly e-mails. Tuesdays at 10 a.m. appears to be the best time to send marketing e-mails. Wednesdays or Thursdays would be your next best option. To get the best results, it is best to avoid Mondays and Fridays. Late morning e-mails seem to receive overall the best open and click-through rates. Alternatively, you might schedule marketing e-mails for 8 p.m. through midnight, 2 p.m. or 6 a.m., as studies show that these are the times when people frequently check e-mail.[12]

---

11 *E-Mail Marketing Field Guide 2018*, Entrepreneur.com.

12 *E-Mail Marketing Field Guide 2018*, Entrepreneur.com.

Subscriber list: This is the list of clients to whom you are choosing to send your marketing e-mails. You can export a list of their e-mail addresses from your customer relationship management (CRM) system and import it into your e-mail marketing account.

List segmenting: You can create different target lists by segmenting your list into smaller groups according to gender, age, and type of procedure or treatment. Once you have added these segments into your e-mail marketing account, you can then send specifically targeted e-mails to the individual groups that would be most interested in that content.

Tracking results: When reviewing campaign results, what trends are you seeing? By monitoring the results, you can learn to make data-driven decisions on content and frequency.

Open rate: This is the percentage of delivered e-mails that were opened by subscribers.

Click-through rate: This is the percentage of delivered e-mails that were opened by subscribers and received at least one click on any link within the e-mail.

Hard bounce error: This means that delivery to the e-mail address has failed, and you should remove that subscriber from your list. Many e-mail marketing software programs will automatically do this for you.

Soft bounce error: This means that an e-mail address is temporarily unavailable but can be kept on your list and tried again later. After several soft bounces, e-mail marketing software will automatically remove the subscriber from your list.

Unsubscribed: This means that the reader of your e-mail no longer wishes to receive e-mails from you. A high unsubscribe rate can also trigger an abuse complaint on your e-mail marketing account.

Abuse complaint: You will usually see this message if more than one of your recipients mark your e-mail as spam. You should aim to keep abuse complaints to a minimum, as over time they can affect your sender rating. In extreme cases, an e-mail marketing company may shut down your account. You might try switching up your e-mail strategy with a softer call to action.

Blogs

Using your monthly cross-promotion as your starting point, integrate twice-monthly written blogs and video blogs (vlogs) in your AMP.

Planning Chart

Action Items to Complete	Who	Date
Monthly cross-promotion: e-mail, post on Facebook & other platforms, update website		
Determine your monthly Facebook giveaway contest prize for the next 12 months		
Determine the subject of your monthly video blogs & written blogs for the next 12 months.		

If your monthly cross-promotion is a free medical-grade sunscreen with injectable filler, you might post a blog article about your sunscreen offerings and another one about fillers. If you have already blogged about these topics before, put a twist on it. For example, you could write about the differences between chemical and physical sunscreens. You could write about the anti-aging properties of hyaluronic acid.

Regular blogging helps to attract new potential clients interested in your services and provides an opportunity for you to stand out as an expert in the aesthetics industry.

Provide value in your content. You achieve this by addressing the questions that both your existing customers and your potential clients have about the aesthetics industry and the services you provide. If people who visit your blog are interested in your content and find value from it, they are more likely to come to you when they are ready to move forward with an aesthetics procedure.

Developing blog content is not as difficult as it might seem. I will share a few ideas to get you started. Your topics are the two services you are cross-promoting this month. Consider the following tips to create engaging titles and content for your blog posts.

- **FAQ blogs:** Keep a list of the questions your patients ask you about the procedures or services you are cross-promoting, and answer each question with a blog post. Stick to the topic at hand, be honest, and provide as much insight as you can.

- **Number blogs:** Top 5 Results from Feminine Health Treatment; 3 Tips for Recovering Faster from Surgery; Top 10 Questions to Ask at Your Consultation.

- **Insider info blogs:** What do you think people really want to know about the industry? Describe a day in the life of your practice. Why is (insert service you are cross-promoting this month) the best solution for (insert problem)?

- **Keyword blogs:** Use SEO to your advantage by focusing your topic around popular search terms. Start by finding keywords related to the service you are highlighting this month.

Now that you have your content ideas, it is time to start writing!

Title: The key to writing a blog title is to think about how the reader would search for the topic online.

Title length: Keep in mind that Google will show only the first 50 to 60 characters of the title in the search results. You can ensure that the most important part of your message is not cut off by tracking your word count using a free online character count tool (https://charactercounttool.com/) or by drafting your title in MS Word.

Search Engine Optimization (SEO): Optimizing content for the search engines means that we are using the right keywords to ensure that our content can be easily scanned and understood by the search engines. This means that our prospective clients, who are searching for our services, will see our listing higher in the search engine results. Keywords should also be written into the body of the blog post in a natural way along with their synonyms and related terms.

Images: Stick to images that are relevant to the blog post. When uploading an image, always aim to add image-alt text, as this allows you to insert keywords and a description of the image to help search engines understand an image's topic.

White space, headlines, and bold font: Leaving some space between paragraphs adds visual appeal to your post. Headlines and bold font break up a lengthy article and keep the reader engaged.

Share buttons: Be sure to add social sharing buttons to your website, so readers can share your content with others. Your web developer should be able to help you add these buttons.

Promoting special offers: At the end of each blog post consider adding an optional promotion. Offers in this section should be relevant to the topic of the post and should not be time-sensitive. This can be a great way to convert the lead! Include a clear call to action (CTA), such as *Click here to book a complimentary consultation*.

Vlogs

Your blog posts can be used as outlines for video scripts. Enlist a staff member to record short video blogs using your mobile phone. A video blog should last no longer than thirty seconds. Most viewers zone out after about ten seconds. Nervous about video blogs? Ease into it by making Boomerangs (a feature on Instagram to make short, fun videos).

YouTube: Upload the video directly to YouTube, making sure to include your keywords in the title and tag them to the video. Embed the video directly into your blog post for search engine optimization.

Social media: When sharing your vlogs to your Facebook Page, we recommend uploading separately to Facebook or Instagram instead of sharing the YouTube link. Uploading your videos directly to Facebook creates a dramatically wider organic reach. You will benefit from Facebook's algorithms, which heavily promote Facebook native video content.

Quarterly Sales Events

We suggest scheduling one event per quarter and outlining the basics for the events in your AMP as follows:

- Body-focused event: Spring
- Face or anti-aging event: Winter/fall
- Feminine health event: Any time of year

- VIP or holiday event with discounts on products and services: Summer/fall

Schedule your event dates for the next twelve months, and select a focus for each event. Choose dates that will allow you to secure the highest participation from your vendors and cooperation from your staff. Evening events typically work best.

Customize your Sales Event schedule according to which treatments or procedures you offer. You might choose to alternate between surgical and non-surgical procedures. For example, your holiday event could highlight product and non-surgical discounts with live demonstrations of injectables and non-invasive body shaping. Perhaps your only elective medical procedure is vaginal rejuvenation, so you will plan for two feminine health events per year.

Action Items to Complete

Event Focus	**Month**	**Date**
Face Anti-Aging		
Body		
Feminine Health or Injectable		
VIP Client Appreciation Event		
Annual One-Day-Only Retail Sale		

Website Updates

Ask yourself the following questions:

1. Who on our staff is responsible for ensuring that the practice website is up to date?

2. Do we have the URL, login, and password for our website?

3. Do we have a web admin to whom we can communicate changes?

4. Do we receive monthly analytic reports regarding our website's performance?

Include a tab on your website for Specials & Events. Add a pop-up on your homepage for specials, sales, and events.

Update your online specials and promotions on a quarterly basis. Show all three of your monthly cross-promotions for the entire quarter on your Specials tab, so people have a resource for current and upcoming specials. Do not forget to put your event information there as well. You can also do a giveaway on your homepage, where people can enter to win a gift certificate worth $1,000 by leaving their contact information. This is a great lead source!

When creating your AMP, do not forget the four essentials:

1. Monthly cross-promotions

2. Social media planning

3. E-mail marketing

4. Quarterly Sales Events

What's Next?

Use the resources provided in this book to build your own AMP and work with your staff to carry out the plan throughout the year. You will soon be on your way to building a more profitable practice and a more loyal client base.

Projected Growth CONSULTING

E-Blasting Checklist

		Who	Due Date	Status
1	Staff to manage e-blasting			
2	Select e-blasting management system			
3	Set up system			
4	Upload patient list			
5	Clean up patient list			
	Create Multiple Lists:			
6	Under 40			
7	Over 40			
8	Male Patients			
9	Surgical Patients			
10	Injectable Patients			
11	Aesthetic Patients			
12	Set up schedule for e-blasting			
13	Set up importing your contact list			
14	Monthly update list from new client report			
15	Add new e-mail inquiries weekly or monthly			
16	Create your graphic campaign in a jpeg			
17	Create marketing plan for subject lines per week			

18	Create your system for weekly topics or type of messaging			
19	Create your campaign			
20	Upload image			
21	Enter subject line			
22	Upload jpeg			
23	Set up your hyperlink to the service page on your website			
24	If not your service page, to set it up to your main URL			
25	Set up your social media hyperlinks			
26	Decide if you want an RSVP button			
27	or a "sign up" opt In button			
28	Enter preview mode			
29	Add yourself and staff to your email list			
30	Run test for staff and yourself first time			
31	If all is good, then...			
32	Verify recipient list			
33	Select Send and Send Now!			
	Suggested Schedule:			
34	**Week 1 Send your Monthly Promotion**			
35	**Week 2 Send your Video Blog for Topic 1**			
36	**Week 3 Send your Facebook Contest of the Month**			
37	**Week 4 Send your Monthly Promotion**			
38	Run your reports by campaign			
39	Review your open rate, opt-out rate and click rate			
40	You are all set to repeat the steps monthly now!			
	PROVEN SYSTEMS CREATE PROVEN RESULTS!			

ProjectedGrowth CONSULTING

1 HOUR MARKETING PLAN

	Action Items to Complete	Who	Due Date	Status
1	Who is the lead for your Annual Marketing Plan & implementation?			
2	Who is in charge of emailing clients weekly?			
3	What day and time will your weekly emails go out?			
4	What email management system will you use?			
5	Who is in charge of deciding on the monthly promotions?			
6	Who will design the monthly promotions?			
7	Who and how will you update you patient email list?			
8	Who is responsible to run the social media contest of the month?			
9	Who is responsible for writing blogs?			
10	Who is responsible to video vlogs?			
11	Who will post blogs and vlogs to your website?			
12	Who will post blogs and vlogs to social media platforms?			
13	Who is in charge of deciding on the quarterly events?			
14	Who is in charge of coordinating the event planning?			
15	Who is in charge of keeping your website updated and current?			
16	Who will review website monthly analytic reports?			
17	Who will manage or review SEO results?			
18	Who will manage or review PPC programs?			
19	Who will run quarterly lead reports by lead type?			
20	Who is in charge of quarterly website functionality reviews?			
21	Who is in charge of keeping website content current?			
22	Who will post social media content weekly to FB and IG?			

23	Who is responsible to run social media reports?			
24	Who is responsible to create the editorial calendar and approve?			
25	Who will upload videos to YouTube?			
26	Who is responsible to comment and reply to social media?			
27	Who will track incoming leads and consultation closing ratios?			
28	Do you need a social media reporting software?			
29	Who will define and implement a Botox Party Program?			
30	Who is responsible for your referral program and rewards?			
31	Do you want to implement a COME back coupon promotion?			
32	Do you want to have a Gift Certificate Drawing on your website?			
33	Do you need to interview a marketing vendor partner?			
34	Do you need to update or get a new website?			
35	Is your current confirmation system working and who is responsible?			
36	What is your highest reaching post to date?			
37	Do you want to boost posts?			
38	Do you want or have patient financing available?			
39	Do you want to explore sales funnels and lead generation?			
40	Who will segment your email list?			
41	What are the top 3 services you want to grow this year?			
42	Who will track the results of contests and promotions?			
43	Who will coordinate with vendors to get free products?			
44	Who will coordinate with vendors for event support?			
45	Who will analyze overall marketing ROI quarterly?			
46	Who is responsible to make changes to improve marketing?			
47	Who is responsible to decide if you need to outsource social?			
48	Do you need social media content? Where will you get it?			
49	What are the biggest challenges for marketing your practice?			
50	Do you need to add staff or restructure positions for these activities?			
	PROVEN SYSTEMS CREATE PROVEN RESULTS!			

PROFIT KILLER #3

3. A LOW-CONVERSION WEBSITE

As the owner of a website, you have a digital salesperson working for you twenty-four hours a day. Your website has a job to attract clients, inform current patients about existing promotions, and create incoming new patient leads. These leads can come by way of e-mail, opt-in on an advertisement, incoming calls, website chat, newsletter opt-ins, gift certificate contests, and online bookings. Whether they came from organic search results, social ads, sales funnels, pay-per-click campaigns, or social media, the goal remains the same: Sales.

Your website often creates a first impression, so strive to create clear calls to action, simple navigation, and a professional look that is visible across devices. Your website is the foundation of your digital marketing strategy, which has replaced traditional methods of marketing in the elective medical industry.

Consider the latest HubSpot 2018 Statistic Report[13]:

- 90% of searchers haven't made up their mind about a brand/business before starting their search.
- 72% of consumers who did a local search visited a business within five miles.
- 28% of searches for something nearby result in a purchase.
- Local searches lead 50% of mobile users to visit stores within one day.

13 The Ultimate List of Marketing Statistics for 2018, HubSpot

When potential clients visit an outdated website, they associate that with the quality of the practice and care. Ensure that your site accurately represents your business. You can differentiate yourself from your competitors with your online imagery. If you have a beautiful office, include office photos or a virtual tour. If you boast a happy staff and team atmosphere, show that with group photos or videos. Determine what makes you unique and/ or your target client type, and construct your website to portray that image.

Your site does not have to be expensive. Many vendors include a new website with their marketing programs. Price options exist for websites under $500 per month, with a new site every two years as part of your contract. Much like your cell phone contract, such a contract assumes that you will need an up-to-date website with new conversion tools and optimization components. Later I will share tips on how to select a good website and digital marketing partner. But before you can find a vendor, it is best to understand the terms, services, and strategies of digital online marketing at a fundamental level.

Studies show that on average, the typical American adult is online over twenty hours a week. Therefore, it is not surprising that over 80% of consumers are searching online for services and providers. Many people use online searching like a phone book, so having your correct information listed is critical.

SEO, or Search-Engine Optimization, determines where your business listing appears to the person searching, and most prospective customers search online first. Many factors can influence this placement and ranking. Your practice needs to show up on the first page for best results from the search engines, especially for the critical services you are marketing. The majority of consumers searching online do not scroll past page one of the search results. Accomplishing this can be approached in a variety of ways and with ranging budgets. We will talk more about that shortly.

Place your business phone number at the top of your website, and verify that it is clickable with click-to-call features enabled. In the course of my work, I have visited hundreds of elective medical sites, and it is rare to find one with an easy-to-find phone number. Do not make it hard for current or future customers to find you. The ideal position for your phone number is the upper right corner on each page placed in a static or fixed position for all of your website pages. This is a quick and inexpensive task to accomplish.

The valuable real estate "above the scroll" should have a Contact Us, click for questions, e-mail us, or a chat option. Studies continue to report that large percentages of online visitors do not scroll down to the lower sections of the pages. The websites of the past with elaborate sliders and a heavy volume of written content are now replaced with sleeker, conversion-based websites with an emphasis on video throughout the site to increase conversion and optimize ranking. This is significant for mobile device use as well.

Your social media links should appear next to the phone number or on the upper border of your website if possible. Many websites have them at the bottom of the page, hoping to incentivize the visitor to consume more information. In actuality, this placement leads people to leave the site and visit a competitor instead. A website requiring fewer clicks and scrolls will convert at a higher ratio. Only have social icon links on your site that you use on a regular basis. It does not look good if your customer or future customer clicks on a social link only to see that you have not updated the profile in months. Be sure to test your social links every month to ensure they work, so your website visitors do not encounter a dead link. **In the cosmetic elective medical industry, Facebook, Instagram, Yelp, YouTube and RealSelf are the most important platforms. RealSelf** can be useful if you use it entirely and offer promotions and post content regularly. **Twitter** is mainly a news source or thought leader platform. **LinkedIn** primarily focuses on professional networking and business collaboration. **Google Maps** is crucial for clients to locate your practice, so double-check that your information is correct and updated if you move your office location.

A mobile-enabled website helps people access your website and information. People conduct the majority of searches on mobile devices. Check your website monthly to make sure your mobile sites function properly. Google now penalizes sites that are not mobile-enabled, which means they do not rank your site as high. Penalties that lower search results are costly and will waste your marketing budget.

The essential pieces of information should be positioned on your website's upper half, which is the most valuable web real estate. Strategically plan out which items will occupy that space. Web visitors to elective medical sites spend the most time reviewing photo galleries and searching for promotions or events. Pay attention to those areas. If you do not have your own "before" and "after" photos, it is okay to use the vendors' "before" and "after" images. However, this is one more of many reasons to treat your staff to free services: It creates an opportunity to take your own authentic "before" and "after" photos, which will ensure a higher level of credibility.

Video content is considered the most critical SEO and marketing strategy to adopt because the majority of searches now are for video content. We will show you how to integrate video as a part of your marketing plan in the chapters about the annual marketing plan and social media strategies. The most popular uses for video are treatment demonstrations, answers to the most commonly asked questions during consultations, patient testimonials, and social media videos that are under one minute. The use of video in the future is a vital part of any online marketing plan and needs to be prioritized.

In addition to desktop and mobile, your website needs to be optimized for digital personal assistants. Digital personal assistants are services like Suri, Alexa, Google Home, or your automobile navigation system. In addition to those, Google

Maps will determine the geographic search parameters, as they are your local business listings and require optimization. Voice command searches, chat assistants, and Google-backed reviews are becoming increasingly more important.

Site engine marketing applies to AdWords or PPC (pay-per-click ads), social paid advertising, sales funnels, crawlers, and cross-linking site-to-site, like Yelp, RealSelf, and other referral sites you may be using.

Pay-per-click, or PPC, is widely used to land your business on page one of your desired search topics. Most consumers do not notice whether the results consist of paid or organic results. Therefore, it is best to have both working for you.

Referral sites, like the laser companies you purchase your devices from, have physician locators. If used correctly, RealSelf and review sites can increase your SEO. These links will increase the conversion of your website.

Short blogs and videos improve conversion ratios and improve your SEO. Blogs are nothing more than short articles. One of the best and inexpensive ways to improve your website's organic ranking is to put new content on your site weekly. Video blogs (vlogs) and blogs are the most efficient way to add content on a weekly basis. Google determines that your site is worthy of being at the top of the search results when new relevant content consistently appears on your website.

The following statistics are from Forbes[14], Impact[15] and other articles regarding the influence of video:

- 75 million people in the U.S. watch videos every day.
- Even the word *video* in an e-mail subject line increases click-through rate by 13%.
- Adding video to e-mails can boost click-through rates by 200-300%.
- Embedding videos in landing pages can increase conversion rates by 80%.
- 90% of customers report that product videos help them make purchasing decisions.
- Nearly 50% of all videos are watched on mobile devices.
- By 2019, internet video traffic will account for 80% of all consumer internet.
- Videos up to two minutes long get the most engagement.
- Internet video will catch up to television in 2019 in terms of hours per day. The study predicts that consumers will watch YouTube for 2.7 hours per day, compared to 2.6 hours of television per day.[16]
- 85% of the US internet audience watches videos online. 45% of those watch more than an hour of Facebook or YouTube videos each week.[17]

14 Video Marketing: The Future Of Content Marketing, Forbes.com
15 *14 Reasons Why You Need to Use Video Content Marketing,* Impactbnd.com
16 7 Digital Marketing Trends That Will Own 2019, Social Report.com
17 37 Staggering Video Marketing Statistics for 2018, WordStream.com

One smart and affordable strategy includes creating your URL or your website address based on popularly searched keywords. Avoid using the practice name or the doctor's last name–especially if it is hard to spell. Do not use popular industry terms that are difficult to spell, such as aesthetics and names of specific technologies, lasers, or procedures. Use keywords that patients will search online to find your services. Those terms are not often a physician's last name or the name of the business. Only searches for widely popular terms will immediately increase your ranking results. You will often notice that microsites and landing pages are named with the city or area where you are located and what you offer, and this is why. Using the two key searchable words of where you are located and what you provide are the components of this strategy. For example, URL addresses like www.medspaseattle.com or www.bodycontouringscottsdale.com are website addresses that will automatically rank higher merely because of the words included.

Patient reviews and testimonials matter to new patients. By adding a testimonial or "praise" page, you will create a selling advantage for your practice. Platforms like Yelp, Google Reviews, and many others contribute ways to garner good reviews. If you are soliciting reviews, systematically utilize them by optimizing and posting them as part of your digital marketing campaign. Many practices accomplish this through their vendor partners and patient database systems.

Your digital marketing strategy includes updating content on your website and across all platforms such as social media, referral sites, and reviews to synergistically improve your online presence. Currently, in this industry, Facebook, Instagram, and YouTube are the social media types creating the highest results for our clients. Consequently, these platforms in that order are where I would recommend you start your social media optimization.

By completing the Website Diagnostic, you can clarify where to focus your efforts. In this chapter, we have shared best practices to create a website that ranks highly and converts visitors into client leads and consultations, as well as strategies and questions to consider when searching for the right strategic digital marketing partner to increase leads and practice revenue.

Here are some things to consider if you want to find a vendor digital marketing partner:

- Do they offer both SEO and SEM with a dashboard tracking system to track ROI?
- Do they have a client base exceeding 100,000 clients?
- Do they optimize platforms for desktop, mobile, and voice command or DPA (digital voice assistant) platforms?
- Are they a Registered Premier Google Partner for your Google-backed reviews?
- Do they optimize for local Google Maps searches?
- Will you receive monthly reporting and strategy analysis with an account manager if you wish?
- Do they have an app to be able to track lead activity?
- Do they specialize in the elective medical industry? View results for the industry with a case study demonstration.
- Look up online reviews and ratings for the company.
- Call a client of theirs to talk about how it is to work with them if you can or wish.
- Allow ninety days to measure results accurately. It will then be necessary to collaborate and tweak the strategies for an additional six months to a year to get the optimum benefit. After that time, if you are not sure, then it is likely that you do not have the right vendor partner. However, when the match is right, it would be foolish to leave.

On the following pages is a website self-diagnostic form for you to use to review your current website and start optimizing your online marketing results.

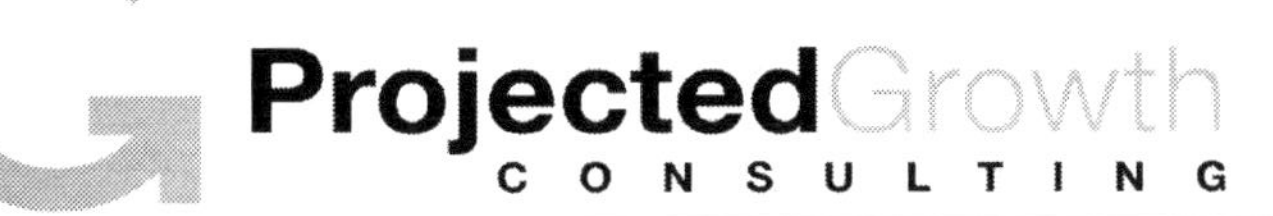

ProjectedGrowth
CONSULTING

	WEBSITE DIAGNOSTIC	**SCORE 1=YES; 0=NO**
1	Is your phone number in the upper righthand corner?	
2	Is your phone number a click-to-call on mobile?	
3	Are your social media icons in the upper page border?	
4	Is your company address easily accessible and fixed to all pages?	
5	Is your phone number large and bold?	
6	Is your phone number in a fixed position on all pages?	
7	Do you have a click-with-questions on your homepage?	
8	Do you have a clickable "Questions" link on the homepage - Links to "Contact Us" form?	
9	Is your clickable "Questions" link in the upper right corner?	
10	Is your clickable "Questions" link fixed to all pages?	
11	Is your "Contact Us" form simple? - only asks for Name, Phone Number and E-mail	
12	Do you have a Blog or Vlog tab?	
13	Do you have a Specials, Promotions, or Events tab?	
14	Do you have a Photo Gallery tab?	
15	Do you have Before and After photos on your site?	
16	Do you have Before and After photos for all services?	
17	Are you taking your own Before and After photos of clients?	
18	Are you posting promotions or events to your website?	
19	Are you posting promotions or events monthly and are they up to date?	
20	Do you post a promotion or event as a pop up on your homepage?	
21	Do you review your monthly Google Analytics report?	
22	Do you currently use pay-per-click, Google Adwords or keywords for traffic?	
23	Does your website URL include what you do and where you are located?	
24	Do you know on average how many leads per month you get from your website?	
25	Do your social media links work?	

26	Do you only have the social media links you actively use?	
27	Do you mirror your Facebook Posts on Instagram?	
28	Do you have a monthly Gift Certificate Contest on your homepage to generate leads?	
29	Do you send out weekly e-mail offers to your clients?	
30	Do you send out any marketing e-mails to your clients?	
31	Do you update your e-mail marketing list monthly?	
32	Do you use MailChimp, Active Campaign or Constant Contact for e-mailing?	
33	Do you review how effective your e-mail marketing campaigns are through analytics?	
34	Do you post 3-5 times per week on Facebook?	
35	Are you posting more than 7 posts per week?	
36	Do you use Insights on Facebook to see how the posts are doing?	
37	Do you analyze your monthly follower trends on social media?	
38	Do you have a goal with your social media posts? EX: SHARE or COMMENT?	
39	Are you successfully growing your social media followers?	
40	Do you use YouTube?	
41	Do you use Instagram?	
42	Do you regularly post vlogs or blogs to your website and social media platforms?	
43	Do you use cross-promotions or value-added offers INSTEAD of discounting?	
44	Do you have a regular process in place to solicit patient reviews?	
45	Do you update testimonials on your website quarterly?	
46	Is your website mobile-enabled?	
47	Do you or staff view your site monthly and on mobile?	
48	Do you get back to e-mail inquiries within 15 minutes - via email or phone?	
49	Do you get back to e-mail inquiries the same day?	
50	Do you have a person responsible or assigned to follow up on e-mail inquiries?	
	Totals	

	BENCHMARKING - How are you doing?	**RANGE**
	WOW - YOU SHOULD TEACH THIS STUFF! CONGRATULATIONS	OVER 25
	AVERAGE - YOU CAN ROCK THIS PRETTY QUICKLY	11 TO 24
	OUCH - YOU NEED TO GIVE SOME ATTENTION ASAP	UNDER 25

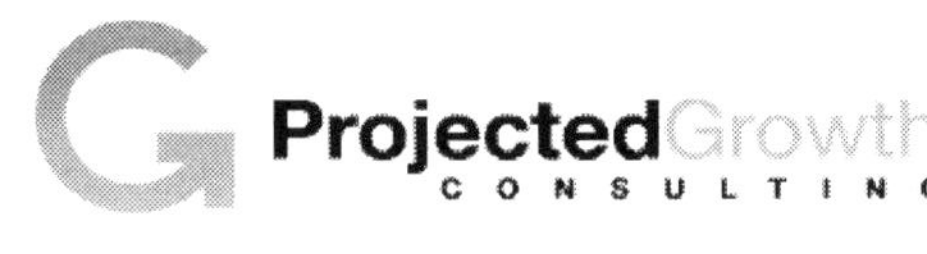

WEBSITE 1 HOUR PLANNING WORKSHEET

	Action Items to Complete	Who	Due Date	Current Status
1	Assign one staff member to lead website vendors			
2	Verify or get practice phone number on top of homepage			
3	Verify or get phone to be click to call			
4	Discuss fixed position for phone number on all pages			
5	Place social links to upper boarder of page			
6	Verify your website is mobile enabled			
7	Visit your website weekly			
8	Visit your mobile site monthly			
9	Assign staff to follow you on all social platforms			
10	Staff to review, upload and update before/afters monthly			
11	Post monthly specials to website quarterly			
12	Post upcoming events to the site 4 weeks before events			
13	Verify or place a Contact Us form field above the fold on all pages			
14	Verify where the incoming email lead inquiries go, which email			
15	Implement a 15 minute response to email inquiries			
16	Test the email inquiry links and status monthly			

17	Review SEO and lead reports monthly			
18	Track expenses by marketing type in a spreadsheet			
19	Set up or verify your process to get patient review			
20	Set up or review your process to post reviews and link on all browsers			
21	Verify all your website links work correctly monthly			
22	Verify that emails to clients link to the correct service highlighted in the promotion			
23	Verify all services are on the site and current, quarterly			
24	Update physician photo to be current, 5 years or newer			
25	Create some short video blogs with Physician or Patient Consultant answering the commonly asked questions			
26	Create clear CALL TO ACTION on your website			
27	Review your SEO strategy			
28	Optimize Blogs and Vlogs with keywords and linking			
29	Review PPC results or look at PPC vendors packages			
30	Create a video content plan for your website			
31	Add a Yelp or other review links to your site if your reviews are good			
32	Mirror FB posts on Instagram			
33	Email your client database weekly -per your Annual Marketing Plan			
34	Create monthly value added promotions for the year			
	PROVEN SYSTEMS CREATE PROVEN RESULTS!			

PROFIT KILLER #4

4. NOT TRACKING KEY METRICS, EXPENSES & BENCHMARKS

After establishing revenue goals by month and measuring weekly performance as outlined in Chapter 1, your practice should experience revenue increases. Next, you will measure expenses monthly and create quarterly cost-cutting strategies for your expense categories. To begin, examine your most significant costs as a *percentage* of income–not simply as dollars spent per month–to see if they are increasing or decreasing. As your company grows and sales increase, your expenses will too. We use percentages because costs are directly related to the desired revenue goals or growing revenue structure. The percentages, however, provide a consistent benchmark to ensure these expenses stay in line with income.

The top five expenses for elective practices include labor, cost of goods, rent, and marketing, then followed by all expenses that exceed 1% of income. These will differ, but they could include supplies, taxes, insurance, etc.

The industry averages for key areas of expenses are as follows:

Marketing	5-20%
Payroll	Under 25%
Owner Draw	5-10%
Net Profit	10-30%
Retail COG	50%
Injectable COG	50%
Retail Average Commission	10%
Cost Per Lead	$100-300

Remember those profit and loss reports we mentioned in Chapter 1? They come into play here as well. Run profit and loss reports for previous years–at least three years back, preferably–and rank them by the highest percentage of income to the lowest. This information helps gauge the health of your practice. Other expense category ranges are listed below.

Insurance	2-3%
Taxes	1-3%
EQ	5-10%
Utilities	.5-1%
Prof. Fees	1-10%

You can examine your fixed costs, but those are more difficult to control or reduce quickly. If they are over 1% of income, you may want to keep them on your radar.

Marketing costs can range widely. Start-up marketing costs for a new practice or new profit center can cost up to 20% while continuing an aggressive increase of market share averages about 10%. To maintain market share, it is recommended that you budget 5% of income toward your marketing strategies.

Rent expense should stay below 5% in most demographics unless you own the building or build a new facility. In these cases the rent is typically offset by renting out some portion of the building to lower this percentage.

A healthy owner draw rate is 5% to 10% for most practice owners and physicians. Creating a set predictable draw is best for the practice. Set the base to a comfortable level that you can receive consistently. If not managed carefully, your practice may struggle to absorb large last-minute draws that affect cash flow and practice credit ratings. Several of our clients have included a bonus for themselves in the weekly revenue calculator for additional motivation – and they keep their percentage private!

The costs of goods for retail and injectable supplies should be 50% or close to it. If that is not the case, then you may have a loss or employee theft issue, or perhaps you are not selling these services at market value. The latter is a direct result of discounting too profoundly.

Most elective medical facilities pay staff a retail sales commission of 10%. They also offer their medical grade skin care and other products at cost for employees. The average product retail cost is approximately $120, and the average retail ticket sale is $250. An essential element for managing retail or product costs is inventory management protocols. When possible, order once per month from vendors in larger quantities to receive volume discounts.

Create clear, written protocols for incoming inventory to be counted and initialed on the packing slip and then entered into inventory. Count and reconcile inventory monthly. If it varies by more than 5%, you will need to count weekly to determine why the discrepancies exist. If, by chance, products are walking out the door, this will most likely solve that issue. Once staff realizes systems and tracking exist, employee theft decreases.

Injectable inventory management is often not monitored and discovered only when these numbers do not add up. To avoid this unpleasant discovery, store these products in locking refrigerators and storage units. The injectable inventory needs to be logged in and out daily, and the manager should be responsible for reconciling the injectable inventory daily. Your job as an owner is to make every effort to create a structured and defined work environment. Eliminating these types of temptations sets everyone up for success!

The retail display should be in the lobby to minimize theft. Alternatively, perhaps put it in locking glass cases or behind the front desk. Since the products are small and expensive, they are easy targets. The placement of your medical retail behind the front desk has another advantage as well: It will increase sales if you implement procedures with your clinician to suggest products to review with clients at checkout.

Spa treatment rooms are another hot spot for theft and profit-impacting losses. If possible, have locking cabinets for back-bar products and supplies, so they are not left in the open while clients are changing before and after treatments.

If you want to create a high-volume retail practice, run retail sales reports by unit quarterly. What are your top twenty sellers? Apply the 80/20 rule. Typically 80% of your volume is coming from sales of 20% of your top-selling products. It may be time to stop carrying the lower-volume retail products. You can special order discontinued products for your clients if needed. Make sure you do not have products that directly compete unless you can clearly explain to staff and patients which product is best for different patient types. Product lines are typically created and built around a few superstar products. When selecting your lines, you can cherry-pick the best or top sellers from different product lines and do not need to carry every product offered for each skin care line.

We recommend carrying a full array of a few lines for your patients who prefer to use one brand. To create a thriving retail inventory, offer various price points of high, medium, and low-priced options. Next, carry products that range from highly active to moderate and all natural or organic options. This approach ensures a variety and full array of retail options for your clientele.

If you are only just starting to offer retail, try placing small opening orders and test the products yourself or create a small patient focus group. Patients love to be invited to participate in these types of programs. Negotiate with your vendor for free travel kits and a few full-size products so you can sell the test kit at a perceived 50% of retail or cost pricing.

When you want to bring on a new line, you can invite ten clients for a discounted offer to try the product line, as well as free laser or peels in exchange for photos documenting the efficacy of the line. Not only does this reduce costs, it provides social proof to increase sales of your new line and other retail as well.

The opposite approach is to put all your apples in one basket. You can drive your rebates up and your costs down by implementing this strategy. By partnering with a few vendors, you will get more samples, on-site training, and event support. Both approaches can be very successful.

Another benefit from having only a few key vendors includes better payment terms, such as ninety days instead of thirty. They may also offer points or rewards for your volume purchases, which can lower your costs. To leverage your vendor benefits, set up quarterly lunch-and-learns for staff, monthly retail sales contests run by the vendor (who will also supply the prize), product collateral, signage, flip books, and selling-scripts for your team.

Vendors can also provide quizzes and certifications during these on-site trainings. Many times, they will help plan an event for the line and come on-site and sell it for you to your patients. For these types of events they can provide catering, treatment visualizers, e-mail content, product bundles, and prizes.

Retail sales goals can be included in your staff compensation plans. Industry standards show that an aesthetician should strive to sell at a 25% retail-to-service ratio. We set these sales goals and see them met on a regular basis. These efforts have longer-term effects as well. In fact, research shows that *"If you sell a client two retail products, there is a 60 percent chance of them returning to the spa or salon. One product, and there is a 30 percent chance of them returning. No product and there's a scant 10 percent chance of them returning."*[18] While some sources differ on the likely-to-return percentage, it generally ranges from 40% to 60%, which is more than worth the effort of pushing those retail products.

---

18 *The Art of Recommendation*, Skindeep Magazine 2018

When I owned my spa, we had a one-to-one ratio goal for facials and met it very often. For your injectors and laser technicians, we suggest a 25% goal of retail sales to services. When you clarify this in a compensation plan, your staff understands the expectations and they can deliver. When we determine these goals, we have found it important to solicit staff feedback about product choices and recommendations. Let them be part of the solution.

For instance, for every $1,000 an injector provides to a client, the goal would be to sell $250 in retail sales. For your aestheticians, the goal would be 50% for facials and 25% for laser treatments. Set up the expectation that each customer will leave with one product. Implement a protocol that has the clinician setting aside a few products for the client to consider at checkout. Front desk staff must also know the benefits and how to sell these products. Offer regular sales training for your team. Lean on your retail vendors to provide quarterly staff lunch-and-learns and product gifts to your team as well.

"Owners and managers track sales as a percentage of retail service dollars. So, if in a pay period, an aesthetician sold $10,000 in services and $2000 in retail sales, his or her retail service dollar would be 20% of retail sales service. Retail is a retention tool. "If a patient leaves the practice with two products that they purchased, they are 40% more likely to come back and see you than if they left with nothing at all," Durocher says. "And clients want products that help them maintain their beauty. I guarantee if a patient is spending $3000.00 on a service plan, [he or she will] spend $700 on skincare to make sure to maintain that service plan."[19]

Staff motivation and net profitability can be linked in a rewarding way for everyone involved. Consider offering a practical bonus plan for your manager or director by rewarding them for cost savings or for driving down percentage costs of goods. They could save on things like office supplies, retail, back bar, medical supplies, and staff turnover.

---

19 *Make your medspa profitable,* The Aesthetic Channel

Once you benchmark your costs of goods by areas, you can set quarterly goals to decrease your expense percentages and create a cost savings split as a bonus to incentivize smarter inventory ordering, sourcing of products, and inventory management of practice supplies under their control. Cost savings bonus structures provide a useful way to save your practice money while rewarding your staff for good work.

Retail success indicates a healthy and profitable practice. It increases patient loyalty and provides an opportunity for staff to make sales commissions. To promote retail, try to have an ongoing special that allows customers to buy two products and receive the third product half off. Clients typically buy one to two products, so you want to encourage that third product sale to, as research suggests, increase the chances they will return. Plus, your clients will likely get the best results by combining the essential treatment elements. Since products last about three months, your client will be back to restock. If a product works well, your patients will notice a difference a few weeks after they stop using it. These active products keep clients coming back. Marketing means getting, maintaining, or growing your patient base, and retail products are essential for protecting, increasing, and maintaining the results for most of the services you offer.

Create a plan to partner with your key vendors and capitalize on your vendor relationships to increase your net profit. Both expense management and vendor selection relate back to your AMP and its effect on increasing your net profit. Share plans for upcoming promotions and events with your vendors before each quarter, and let them support your campaigns with products, staff training, and client appreciation gifts-with-purchase programs. Engaging your vendors to increase net profit this way could be its own section. Briefly, however, these main strategies can get you started.

An essential vendor partnership is the one with our injectable companies. Many practices do not realize that you can often treat staff for free with your sales rep's assistance. Ask for free products to reward new or existing staff. Vendors can supply products for training sessions as well. Often they can provide products to cover your cross-promotion of the month. Implement set quarterly meetings with your vendor partners in your AMP. During those vendor meetings, share your upcoming promotions, contest of the month prizes, and event calendar to receive the most help from them. You can set sales goals with them to grow your injectable services, so it is worth their time and resources to provide you with these benefits.

Although you will track your sales weekly to reach your monthly goals, you want to review expenses only on a quarterly basis. When you are working to increase revenue, you can measure it immediately and see a difference. If you look at your expenses in relation to sales too often, the slower pace to improve upon spending may discourage you. If you change a vendor or find better pricing on supplies, results will show up a few months after you have made those changes. Be patient. Small incremental adjustments will begin to show. After a year of taking these steps, you will be pleased with your progress.

Complete the 1 Hour Expense Reduction Action Worksheet on the following pages to prioritize the steps to improve your net profitability. You can review your practice diagnostic from the beginning of the book and focus on the financial section for areas to consider targeting. After listing the areas of concern, assign them to the appropriate team member and define a due date and time frame for the projects. Set up quarterly meetings now to measure your effectiveness, edit your action list, and celebrate your progress. Continue to review the numbers monthly and then benchmark your percentages quarterly to see if things are moving in the right direction. If they are, continue on the same path. If they are not, create another strategy with your team or reach out to us for additional help.

ProjectedGrowth CONSULTING

1 HOUR EXPENSE REDUCTION PLAN

	Action Items to Complete	Who	Due Date	Status
1	Fill out the benchmarking and diagnostic forms			
2	Run your profit and losses with percent of income			
3	Look at the major categories of expenses first.			
4	Payroll			
5	Marketing			
6	Rent			
7	Owners Draw			
8	Retail COG			
9	Injectable COG			
	Surgical COG			
10	Net profit percentage			
11	Any other expenses over 1% of Income			
12	Review these percentages to last years percentages			
13	Note which percentages have gone up.			
14	If you haven't already do your Revenue Planning Sheets			
15	Look at revenue this year to last year by month			
16	Has the income gone up or down by month?			
17	Note which percentages have gone up as a percent of income.			
18	Can they be justified.			
19	Is your retail cost of goods 50% or retail sales or under?			
20	Is your injectable cost of goods 50% or under injectable sales?			

21	Is your monthly inventory over or under counts?			
22	Set up process to manage inventory and supplies			
23	Review and adjust inventory			
24	Set up quarterly goals for expense savings			
25	Set 3 expense saving goals per quarter - at the most			
26	Review results monthly, it takes 3 months to see changes			
27	Look at labor saving options			
28	Is staff creating enough revenue to support compensation plan?			
29	Mid levels should create 4x their total cost to the company.			
30	Providers should create 5-7X their total costs to the to the company.			
31	Rewrite comp plans if necessary with new sales thresholds.			
32	If labor is up significantly set up performance reviews.			
33	Review job descriptions for each staff member.			
34	Consider a bonus for costs savings for manager.			
35	Clarify expected cost ratios by department and service.			
36	Work with vendors to drive down costs with bulk orders.			
37	Plan with vendors for complimentary products for promotions.			
38	Set up a sales event.			
39	Start utilizing the Annual Marketing Plan process.			
40	Review retail and reduce products to top sellers.			
41	Set up quarterly and monthly steps to meet your goals			
42	Break down to departmental and weekly action items			
43	Set up monthly management meetings			
44	Schedule quarterly half day session for management			
45	Implement regular staff meetings			
	PROVEN SYSTEMS CREATE PROVEN RESULTS!			

PROFIT KILLER #5

5. NOT IDENTIFYING KEY PERFORMANCE INDICATORS AND MARKETING ROI

Key Performance Indicators (KPIs) are defined in this book as the number of leads, conversions, and consultation ratios combined with the Return On Investment (ROI) necessary to create the desired revenue or sales for your practice.

We recommend forecasting revenue at least one year out with a reasonable growth percentage based on past service sales, marketing budget, staffing providers, and facility capacity. Revenue projections need to be based on realistic and measurable goals and strategies. In order to get staff support, these goals should be broken down by services per week or month and based on past performance. Practices cannot grow magically without a change from doing business as usual. This is the primary reason that teams often do not support or work toward corporate key initiatives or projections.

As mentioned earlier, your marketing strategy primarily relies on digital marketing. I often hear questions from practice owners wondering if their marketing efforts work or not. Measuring your performance will provide you with confidence that you are investing marketing dollars wisely. And, you will know if you are not spending them wisely and have the knowledge to make adjustments.

To measure performance, create a list of each marketing effort used for your practice. The goal is to get a 4:1 return or a 400% ROI. In other words, for every $1,000 spent on marketing, your practice should make $4,000 in revenue. In this chapter, we will share how to measure and analyze your current marketing efforts.

Below is a sample of our ROI and KPI Worksheet. You can download an electronic or printable version of this form in the Resources Files at the end of the book.

Begin by reviewing the past three years of total sales.

Revenue Total	Annual Total	Mo Ave
2019 YTD		
2018		$ -
2017		$ -

The most common digital marketing strategies fall into the following categories:

1. Website
2. SEO
3. PPC
4. Sales funnels
5. Social media management
6. Social media paid advertising
7. Referral sites like RealSelf
8. Other free physician locators

These are listed in the order of importance to guide you in your budget-planning efforts.

First, enter your marketing spending into the worksheet below. Specify the number of leads coming through your website and the quantity of leads coming into the practice via your various marketing channels. Even if you do not track from lead to revenue, you can review overall marketing expenditures versus the number of consultations to arrive at a benchmark cost-per-lead estimation. You will want to find out the following:

- How many leads do you get?
- How many consultations do you perform?
- How many cases are booked?
- What is your revenue, which leads us to your estimated ROI?

Number of Leads per Year	2019 YTD	2018	2017	2013	Annual Budget
Organic SEO Website Inquiries					
Pay Per Click Leads Website					
Social Media					
Real Self					
Physician Locator Website					
Radio					
TV					
Print					
Billboards					
Patient or Staff Referrals					
Physician Referrals					
Paid Social Lead Adv's					
Total					

Other KPIs to measure include call conversion, lead response time, and consultation closing ratios. If you are not currently tracking them, start now. From the Resource Chapter of this book, you can download free forms to start tracking and measuring.

Practice Statistics	2019 YTD	2018	2017
Number of Consultations			
Number of Surgeries perfomed			
Number of Injectable Appointments			
Injectable Cost for the period			
Retail Cost of Goods for the period			
Medical Grade Retail Sales Revenue			
Number of Aesthetic Appointments			

In the aesthetics industry, it costs $100 to $300 to get a new client call or e-mail inquiry. For existing clients, your receptionist, front desk staff, and patient consultants have most of the impact by way of customer service skills and benefit selling training. In fact, "*Existing customers spend 67% more than new customers.*"[20] Your receptionist plays an important role in new client conversions and upselling or cross-selling at check-in or checkout. Since "*customer service stats show that new customers cost anywhere between 5 and 25 times more expensive than retaining existing customers,*" your receptionist can play an important role in helping you retain and grow clients through additional sales.[21]

Every marketing dollar spent has a job: To create a call or inquiry online. Therefore, lead costs should be tracked. Conversion ratios affect your KPIs and how to budget for the sales and revenue goals that you are aiming to hit. If you do not track your KPIs, you cannot know what corrections to make to adjust your course.

---

20 *Customer Loyalty: The Ultimate Guide*, HubSpot
21 *The Value of Keeping the Right Customers*, Harvard Business Review

Social Media Statistics	2019 YTD	2018	2017
Facebook - Followers			
Facebook - Highest Number of Comments			
Facebook - Highest Number of Shares			
Facebook - Highest Organic Reach			
Instagram			
Patient E Mail List			
YouTube			

The cascade is as follows: Cost per lead, conversion ratio, show-up rate, consultation closing ratio, and client retention with the average cost per lead of $100 to $300 mentioned previously.

The lead conversion rate varies by lead type. While pay-per-click should convert at 25% from inquiry to consultation, the conversion ratio from social media paid advertising or sales funnel campaigns and landing pages convert at approximately 10%. The actual rate depends upon your response time and pre-constructed funnels and e-mail drip campaigns. The cost per lead is lower in the social media paid advertising arena, but the conversion ratios are equally lower. Even though you get more leads from a social media-based funnel, the quality of those leads seems to convert at the same rate of $100 to $300 in terms of the cost to get a new consultation in the door.

The average consultation-closing ratio is around 30%. Your goal should be 50%, which is realistic and attainable when done properly. A highly successful practice may reach 75%. We measure all metrics on this for our event programs. Last year we sold over $18 million for our clients at our on-site Sales Events. When the RSVP goal of thirty people is met, about 20 to 22 people attend, which results in a 76% purchase rate. When practices believe they have higher than 80% closing ratios, we typically find that they are not tracking these numbers.

- If you are closing under 25%, you need immediate training and protocol changes.

- If you are closing 50% of your consultations, you are doing several things correctly and have room for improvement.

- If you can achieve 75% or better when closely measuring, you are performing at a top level. If this is the case, it is time to spend more money on lead generation and training another patient consultant for your practice, because you are firing on all cylinders!

The percentage of medical denials and financing-declined patients at our events is less than 10%. If you believe your closing ratio deficit is due to those issues, you may want to take a closer look. When a potential client is not confident or comfortable with a practice, the easiest excuse is the surprise of the cost or the lack of financing. If this is occurring at a rate exceeding 10%, you may want to analyze customer service, facility condition, and staffing for clarity. This would be a good time to hire a secret shopper or friend to pose as a potential client to find out the actual reasons for these ratios. Even if you get the worst news, at least you find out what you need to improve or change to grow your practice.

Let us put this into perspective. If you spend $3,000 per month on a PPC campaign, you should expect 10 to 30 leads with a consultation-booking ratio of 25% or better. As an example, let us say you get twenty-five leads, which end up being twelve consultations and six booked cases. If the average case is $4,000, then the sales are $24,000. To maintain the 4:1 ROI, our goal would be to exceed revenue of $12,000 in booked cases. In other words, this budget could have supported a sale as low as $2,000 per procedure with these conversion statistics. This campaign qualifies as a good ROI.

The less measurable portion is the ongoing repeat volume and retail purchases from these clients–not to mention the ability to continue to market to the leads that did not come in for consultations. It is likely that 20 to 30 people will contact the office via phone or online channels–all of them excellent leads to whom the practice can continue to market and promote services in hopes of eventually converting them into paying clients. When the clients opt in for a social media advertisement or e-mail about an event or special, they are added to your marketing database to continue to nurture them until they become ready to buy. Make sure to set up a process to add all new potential patient leads to your patient e-mail database or do this automatically via click funnels or whichever system is being utilized for lead generation and sales-funnel campaigns. The goal for marketing is to maintain top-of-mind awareness so that when this client is ready to buy, they think of your practice.

Let us consider that same budget for sales-funnel landing pages. For the same $3,000 investment, we would anticipate 200 to 300 leads at a 10% conversion ratio. This puts us right back in the 20 to 30 lead range. Now you have the benefit of having the e-mails addresses of all 200 to 300 leads to continue to automate drip content and court them into making an appointment or a consultation. This is an excellent way to quickly build a large target or lead list of potential patients. A new practice can utilize this method to quickly create a quality local marketing list over six to twelve months.

Depending on your vendor partners or scheduling software programs, you can easily track conversion ratios with standard reporting. Although you will need to enter some of your business data, consider this dashboard and reporting as value-added services when looking for website, lead generation, or marketing partners. Measuring your ROI from these expenditures can either keep you up at night or make you feel confident in your investments. You must know what to ask for regarding this information. Often, practices are so excited by the pure number of leads that they feel like they have made a wise marketing investment. Beware if your vendor does not provide a dashboard and monthly tracking reports to analyze your results. Some options out there create a high number of low-quality leads to create the illusion of a high ROI. In short, you must be able to measure the performance and ROI on your marketing investments to feel confident you have made a wise investment. If you have the information required to make that assessment, then you are most likely looking at a good, reliable marketing partner.

ProjectedGrowth CONSULTING

1 HOUR KPI & ROI PLAN

	Action Items to Complete	Who	Due Date	Status
1	Complete Revenue Planning Worksheet			
2	Complete Marketing ROI Form			
3	Run profit and loss for last year - detailed with % of Inc			
4	Identify the marketing vendors by name			
5	Look at average spend per month			
6	Run a report of your monthly sales			
7	Figure out your average monthly revenue			
8	Identify how many appointments you need per week by profit center to make facility sales goals			
9	Take that number and double it to calculate number of consults needed per week			
	How are you doing? Over or Under			
10	Take the number consults needs times 4 to calculate desired number of leads per week.			
11	Calculate from these your KPI's for the following:			
12	How many leads per month do you need?			
13	How many consultations per month do you need?			
14	What is your current closing ratio?			
15	What is your current phone conversion ratio?			
16	How many leads are coming in through each lead source?			
17	Patient referrals?			
18	On line: website, email, ppc, social paid adv			

19	Are you getting a 4X ROI on marketing dollars spent?			
20	Set up or review your tracking for call conversion monthly			
21	Set up or review your reporting for closing ratios monthly			
22	Review monthly lead reports for all lead sources			
23	Calculate cost per lead and ROI for all lead sources			
24	Research changing marketing per your results			
25	Set up group bonus structure after setting monthly goals			
26	Train staff with the consultation protocol			
27	Utilize your Weekly Revenue Tracker			
28	Clean up your e-mailing list			
29	Sub-divide your list and make it segmented			
30	E-mail weekly according to plan			
31	Implement Facebook contest of the month			
32	Utilize the entries as a lead source			
33	Specify sales event months and services			
34	Pull your lead tracking reports - weekly			
35	Set up tracking for call conversion - weekly			
36	Set up reporting for closing ratios - weekly			
37	Review monthly lead reports for all lead sources			
38	Calculate cost per lead and ROI for all lead sources			
39	Research changing marketing per your results			
40	Set up group bonus structure after setting monthly goals			
41	Train staff with the consultation protocol			
42	Look at labor saving options			
43	Review compensation plans for each staff member			
44	Create the three main goals for the year			
45	Set up quarterly and monthly steps to meet your goals			
	PROVEN SYSTEMS CREATE PROVEN RESULTS!			

PROFIT KILLER #6

6. THE INABILITY TO CONVERT EXPENSIVE LEADS

"Although your customers won't love you if you give bad service, your competitors will." - Kate Zabriskie, Founder of Business Training Works

Lead conversion is the ability to transfer a caller, a patient question at the front desk, an e-mail, or online lead into an appointment or a consultation, which is required for the financial success of any aesthetic practice. No marketing budget is large enough if your team cannot convert those leads into appointments.

This chapter shares proven techniques we teach and use on behalf of our clients every day to beat industry conversion averages. Would your business not benefit from a highly skilled receptionist and front desk team with the skills necessary to convert your leads at high ratios? For elective medical practices, the receptionist performance can account for 25% of the practice revenue, and *"70% of the customer's [buying] journey is dictated by how the customer feels they are being treated."*[22] The front desk's effect on revenue is more visible when the team is not very skilled at marketing or sales because owners likely notice lower revenue. However, front desk staff is usually not noticed as much when they perform well.

The ideal front desk person, patient consultant, and receptionist must love people, and that personality trait cannot be taught. Make sure you are hiring for attitude and training for skill. After all, according to Salesforce, *"55% of customers are willing to spend more money with a company that guarantees them a satisfying experience."*[23] As the owner, your responsibility is to put the right

---

22 *70% of Buying Experiences are Based on How the Customer Feels They are Being Treated*, Industry Analyst Inc

23 *Customer Service Stats: 55% of Consumers Would Pay More for a Better Service Experience*, Salesforce.com

staff into positions that suit your practice and their personality. The people who will be successful at these jobs are motivated to over-perform and delight your customers. They find pleasure in delivering a high level of customer service. When you can get this personality type at your front desk and in the consultation portion of your business, the results will be self-evident.

An established greeting protocol can welcome customers and new clients. Guiding the call well creates a high level of confidence and the WOW factor necessary to convert your potential patient. With 70% of buying experiences *"based on the emotional experience of the customer and how he or she feels she is being treated,"*[24] you want to be sure to treat them all well.

You want to make the experience easy. Take customers by the virtual hand. A clear greeting script and protocol will transform the conversion ratios at the front desk. This can be simple.

Option 1:

> "Hello, this is Tracey. Thank you for calling Aesthetic Cosmetic Surgery. How can I help you today?"

Option 2:

> "Thank you for calling Aesthetic Cosmetic Surgery. This is Tracey, how can I help you?"

Be clear and direct with your script. Take the time to format this and have it in writing. Consistently use the script so anyone covering the front desk knows what to say. These small details affect the level of professionalism and customer service of your business.

---

24 7 Ways Consumer Support Affects Your Bottom Line, Talkdesk.com

The next process is converting the call to an appointment or consultation. Talkdesk points out that *"70% of U.S. consumers are willing to spend more money to go with a company who they believe will provide top-notch service."*[25] This often begins with the initial phone call and the use of a consistent script. You can direct the customer down the right path only if you know where you are trying to lead them. The reception position often pays less than other jobs or is considered entry level, so it is often not credited with the importance it deserves. Keep in mind that *"78% of consumers have bailed on a purchase that they intended to make because of poor customer service."*[26] If you lack good receptionist protocols and staffing, it can cost thousands of dollars by killing expensive leads every single day.

If the goal is to book an appointment, then proceed by offering two days that work for the office calendar.

Example:

Office: Would Tuesday or Friday be better for you?

Client: Tuesday.

Office: Wonderful, do you prefer morning or afternoon?

This simple process efficiently guides the call. This act alone will save time and increase conversion.

By the way, you want to appear busy while making them a priority. Maybe you just opened and can book them anytime, but you do not want to tell them that. The client will be suspicious if they can get in today or know you do not have many appointments on the books. You need to guide the call as above with option A or option B. People want to go to a busy, thriving practice and not

25 7 Ways Consumer Support Affects Your Bottom Line, Talkdesk.com
26 7 Ways Consumer Support Affects Your Bottom Line, Talkdesk.com

one desperate for clients. Most people love to go to the new hip restaurant even when there is a waitlist for weeks, and they might even be waiting for hours once they arrive. People assume that the restaurant must be good if it is busy and has a wait list.

Benefit selling, which is the preferred method for a high customer service and consultative experience, takes preparation. If the caller has questions about a service, we ask them what result they are looking for. Hence benefit selling. If the phones are too busy to take the necessary uninterrupted time with the caller, have an expert or consultant on your staff return the call within fifteen minutes or transfer the call to them and away from the busy front desk.

Write down your stories about a patient, a co-worker or even yourself that explain why you like these services. If staff is not allowed to get free services, they can share the experience of a patient without using the patient's name. They can talk about how impressed they were with the patient's results and how exciting it is to watch these transformations. As a past med spa owner myself, I recommend spending money to allow staff to experience your products and services as a worthwhile marketing expense. Happy internal customers will create a culture that requires less management time, money, correction, and complaint resolution. Let your staff speak from experience if possible. You know the popular saying: "Stories are sharing and telling is selling."

What if the incoming caller asks for pricing? Perhaps the caller requests a service by name that you do not offer. This is where benefit-selling training is critical. Your receptionist should know the range of costs and how to suggest another technology in place of the one being requested. Ideally, they have been trained to know the various names of toxins or non-invasive fat reduction. The best way to do this is to make a list of all the services you offer, list the other names of services and products treating the concern, and lastly list the price range for the services. This material should be reviewed and memorized–or at least referenced in writing–at the front desk. If a call comes in requesting CoolSculpting®, and you do not offer it, the next step is to explain that CoolSculpting®

reduces fat non-surgically in spot treatment areas and ask them which areas concern them. Next, explain that you have an alternative treatment to address unwanted fat, and identify the benefits to your service compared to the one they called about. Perhaps your service is more comfortable, less expensive, or a newer option. This knowledge keeps the leads coming your way. Reference the Benefit Selling Cheat Sheet in the Reference Chapter of the book for the most common elective services offered.

Be efficient and ready to lead the call. Building rapport can be easy if you are able to listen and converse because you are prepared and know all about the services. These phone scripts and conversion protocols will grow your practice's monthly revenue in a measurable way. If you own or manage an elective medical practice, it is essential to learn how to convert leads at the highest possible rate.

Assuming your goal is to book a consultation, you need to tell the patient why it will be a benefit to them. Many clients book these elective medical appointments like they would a manicure or pedicure appointment, without understanding the need for a consultation prior to treatment. They do not always realize that misplaced BOTOX® can cause ptosis for three months and leave them looking like they have had a mini-stroke, or that they can get a painful burn or a permanent lack of pigment from a laser treatment. We want to explain nicely why the consultation benefits them. I suggest a script like this:

During your consultation, you will see the doctor. Please bring any pictures or questions to discuss during our time together. We want to make sure you are selecting the best service to give you the results you are looking for within your budget and recovery time frame, and that it is a medically safe option for you. We offer this benefit of a consultation because we know how important it is for you to know your options and the possible downsides and recovery times for some of these treatments. We also find that we offer some solutions that you might not realize can enhance or create the results you are looking for. An educated client is our best client. Let us see where we can fit you in right away.

Be sure to explain what the consultation will entail and what they can expect. Suggest that they do research online about the service if they have not done so already. Guide them to your website or perhaps RealSelf so they prepare their questions or concerns. You might use this script:

This time is for you! You will have Dr. Jones and Mary all to yourself. They know all the secret ways to make you look and feel your absolute best. I am so excited to have you come in and meet with us, and I will get to meet you in person then. You are really going to love this spa and the staff here. I really enjoy my team and working here. Did you have any questions for me?

This kind of passion is contagious and will help your clients feel welcome and comfortable.

Every office needs a protocol for appointment confirmation. It might seem simple, but it is easily overlooked. People are busy and forget things midstream. You need to confirm appointments, create your own protocol, and have it in writing. This process can be automated. However, it still needs to be assigned to a staff member as part of their job description. A text opt-in is fine a few days prior, yet a same-day reminder is necessary in the morning. For online bookings, a call is preferred to qualify and increase the likelihood that your appointment will show up.

When I speak to a potential client, most of them believe more leads would fix their financial challenges. Although this is sometimes true, more often the issue concerns a low conversion ratio of leads to appointments or consultations. Unless you measure and track the number of leads coming in per month versus the number of those that book, you may not be aware of this challenge. As a result, you might keep spending more money on marketing to create an increase in lead volume. Obviously, that will not fix the problem no matter how much you spend.

Many practices struggle to get enough leads, convert them into consultations and close consultations at a high rate. Once you convert the leads into paying customers, you want to keep them. *"Because retaining an existing customer costs significantly less, both in terms of marketing and maintenance, than landing a new one. Additionally, repeat customers are more likely to spend more money on each purchase. So, if you want to make sure your profits are hearty and your retention rates are high, you must provide amazing customer service."*[27]

Your work in this area will pay rewards over time. Even *"increasing customer retention rates by 5%" can increase "profits anywhere from 25% to 95%."*[28]

Over 90% of customers who are dissatisfied with your customer service experience will, rather than telling you if something is wrong and how you can improve it, just not come back. Therefore, it's in your best interest to provide consistently high quality support services to help increase your retention rate and improve your bottom line."[29]

Only about 4% of dissatisfied customers let the company know that they are unhappy with their service.[30]

Our business consulting clients typically come to us with one of three problems:

- Not having enough leads,
- struggling to convert the leads to appointments, or
- closing their consultations.

27 7 Ways Consumer Support Affects Your Bottom Line, Talkdesk.com
28 *Prescription for cutting costs*, Bain & Company Inc
29 7 Ways Consumer Support Affects Your Bottom Line, Talkdesk.com
30 7 Ways Consumer Support Affects Your Bottom Line, Talkdesk.com

Often, they experience problems in all three areas. To review, the average cost per lead in the elective medical industry is $100 to $300 for pay-per-click advertising, and the typical budget for that is about $2,000 to $3,000 per month. Typically, this budget yields 20 to 30 leads per month on average. For this lead source, 25% of the leads should convert to appointments or consultations, and the consultations should close at 50% or better. Therefore, the KPIs for a PPC budget of $3,000 per month translates into thirty leads, seven to eight consultations, and three to four booked cases. Then you take the average revenue per service advertised. If it is body contouring at $3,000 per case, the revenue produced is $12,000 if four cases are booked. This means you spent $3,000 in marketing for this campaign and sold $12,000. That is a 25% cost of marketing or a 4X ROI. This amount reaches the minimum sales required to make this a good investment.

The average landing page for social media as a funnel approach costs approximately $2,500 to $4,000 per month and results in 60 to 120 leads. If this is your marketing strategy, the Key Profit Indicators, or KPIs, would be that out of the 100 leads, fifteen will book an appointment. If you are going to spend money to make the phone ring, then make sure your staff is ready and trained to convert those leads. The front desk staff and reception team cannot be underestimated or over-trained. A front desk team can make or break an aesthetic practice. This training needs to be offered quarterly. Online virtual options are an affordable way to keep your staff at their best or to fill in training gaps due to turnover or movement within the practice.

The key industry benchmarks that apply to the first part of the sales process called lead conversion are response time, responses necessary, and booking conversions to appointment or consultation. The quicker your response, the higher your conversion ratio. If you respond to people via text or e-mail, try to do so within fifteen minutes. Incoming new patient calls should convert at 25% or better, so a 1:4 ratio. Online leads should convert between 10% and 20% or 1 to 2 out of 10. Once you start tracking how you are doing, you can adjust your lead-generation sources to create the desired number of cases for your practice or provide more conversion training or support to your staff. But first you need to know the desired number of cases by completing your Revenue Plan, which we discussed in Chapter 1. If you have not completed your Revenue Plan, now is a good time to pause and finish that before proceeding.

The goal is to convert any lead type or incoming response into a phone conversation. Text and e-mail are a close second. Again, response time cannot be underestimated, and respond back using the method they prefer. For online leads, we use The Rule of Two: two voice-mails, two texts, and two e-mails. After that, leave them in the funnel and let the funnel do its job. Over time, they may convert into a new patient. We do not advise continuing to call and text them if they do not respond after those attempts. Social media and online leads are not as serious as an incoming phone call or e-mail inquiry requesting information or opting into your offer. Do not stalk your leads. Patients smell desperation and will be gone for good if you irritate them. But you can continue to drip on them automatically through your sales funnel. If you do not have a funnel set up, simply add them to your e-mail list to stay in touch so they will reach out to you when ready. Regarding these online leads and The Rule of Two, we suggest the following front desk protocol:

- Start with a phone call and leave a nice scripted voice-mail within fifteen minutes of getting the lead.
- 30 minutes later, send a text.
- 30 minutes after that, send an e-mail.
- Do that immediately after getting the lead, and then once again before the end of the day.

Try your best. But if this does not get a response, let them go. You have given it a good try! And remember: At the end of the day, this is a numbers game.

A common belief is that clients are price shopping or calling all your competitors. If your front desk does their job, the prospective patient will not make the next call to your competitor. They are waiting to be WOWED. Your job is to lead them seamlessly through the decision tree and book them. They do not have time to call around or do multiple consultations. But they will do it if they do not get a good feeling on the call or an answer to their concerns. When they run into a well-trained receptionist, they do not stray far from your practice. Follow these steps whether you are a receptionist, patient consultant, or owner. You need this skill. A positive customer experience helps you keep and grow your patient base–and a profitable, sustainable business.

Track your KPIs in order to identify where you can improve.

- Are you getting enough leads?
- Are they taking the opt-in offer?
- What percentage are showing up?

You need to track this for 30 to 90 days so you can continue to tweak and improve your process and offers. You cannot improve what you cannot measure. And think about what is in it for them. Your offers and promotions need to be too good to resist. If necessary, a deposit or a credit card reservation can reduce your no-shows, but it is also a barrier to entry and can drive conversions down. Therefore, do not implement this unless it is deemed necessary from the ratio statistics collected over the 30 to 90 days period.

You can incorporate a lot of ways to improve conversion, and one involves video. Create welcome and confirmation videos and another for commonly asked questions about your services. Use them as part of your e-mail confirmation and nurturing structure. Do not underestimate the power of human touch–even by video–to nurture lead conversion to the highest industry averages.

Use your lead dashboard or CRM to track conversions and necessary follow-up actions. If you need tracking forms, you can download them from the Resource Chapter in the back of this book. Tracking, benchmarking, and reporting are your navigation systems and can help you move from good to great. Use them to measure lead conversion and closing ratios. These ratios are invaluable for your decision-making regarding marketing budgets, funnel strategies, and necessary training to grow practice revenue. You can use this information to tweak offers and to determine if more training is necessary to bring performance up to industry averages.

Call and lead conversions are the first steps in the sales process. If you have the leads, that is great. Let us not waste them. Implement a lead conversion process that builds rapport with benefit selling techniques. It is time to beat the industry averages. You can rise above the competition and increase your profitability with these strategies.

ProjectedGrowth
CONSULTING

1 HOUR CONVERSION PLAN

	Action Items to Complete	Who	Due Date	Status
1	Review the basics - Answer by second ring			
2	On hold no more than one time			
3	Move calls off the front desk to convert to consultation			
4	Smile--they can hear your smile!			
5	Create greeting protocol for all to utilize			
6	Update and review your on-hold script			
7	Incorporate your monthly special into greeting or closing			
8	Lead the call			
9	Offer the consult day and time option - assume the close			
10	Ask what results they are looking for			
11	Then explain the benefits of the service - and if they match			
12	Review the consultation structure with the team			
13	Practice explaining the consultation process on the phone			
14	Explain they will get time with the Dr. at the consultation			
15	Create your BEST service - suggest research prior to consultation			
16	Recommend your website for more information or photo gallery			
17	Ask if they would like you to email them more information			
18	Track number of new client calls			

19	Track number of consultations booked			
20	This will give you your monthly conversion ratio			
21	The goal is over 50%			
22	You have one chance to WOW them...make it good!			
23	It costs \$100 to \$300 to make the phone ring!			
24	Allow one hour for your consultation			
25	Agree on the process and roles with your entire team			
26	Practice credentialing your providers!			
27	Also, practice your 30 second credentialing of yourself!			
28	What makes our practice special or unique			
29	Share your personal experiences of getting services if you can			
30	Practice building rapport and open-ended questions			
31	Review service benefits selling sheet			
32	Role play at weekly meetings			
33	Have a contest to see who can convert the most!			
34	Practice educating clients on why they should want the proper credentialed provider and the downsides of potential bad outcomes			
35	Know current specials, events and contests.			
36	Try to experience services and products and share			
37	Listen more than you talk			
38	Make the patient excited to meet you when they come in			
39	Have fun! It is contagious.			
40	Ask for more training if you need it.			
	PROVEN SYSTEMS CREATE PROVEN RESULTS!			

PROFIT KILLER #7

7. UNDEFINED CONSULTATION STRUCTURE & TRACKING TOOLS

Once you have learned how to turn leads into appointments, the next step is closing the sale in a consultation. Many practitioners make the mistake of "winging" this part of the process. We have found that a defined consultation structure helps many of our clients raise patient closing ratios and provide more consistent results.

Because we have hosted over 2,000 on-site Sales Events, we have a great deal of consultation and closing experience. During these events, we do a series of fifteen-minute consultations and close at least ten cases in less than two hours. Below we will outline how to do a high closing consultation in your office, which differs from the shortened event consultations. This is because at the events, we do an educational consultation in a group format, followed by personal mini-exams to review health history and pricing with the patient and physician. The definition of a successful closed consultation is that the doctor and patient agree on a treatment for the desired results and a deposit is taken. The same principles apply in the office for regular consultations as they do at the events. The average closing ratio at our on-site events is 76%. Your in-office consultations can be just as good or better.

In order to exceed a closing ratio of 70% or above, you must allow time for the process to work. While you may be tempted to "play the numbers game" by cramming as many consultations as possible into your schedule, this can hurt your sales. A comprehensive in-office consultation takes time. The patient should never feel rushed as you listen to their needs, address any concerns, and gently guide them through the process of deciding on the appropriate treatment. We recommend scheduling at least an hour for each consultation. This will give you time to build rapport and discuss treatment options, budget, and recovery times. For new clients, this will be their first live impression of your practice. You want them to walk away impressed with the advice they received and confident they are making an informed decision. Helping patients understand all the options available, along with the associated costs and risks, will prevent regrets or confusion later.

The consultation should determine the best treatment for the patient, and an effective one builds trust and credibility between patient and practice. Whoever conducts the process needs to be prepared with practical knowledge and ways to help your clients feel relaxed. Your client does not want a robot reading procedures from a list. Have a few stories to accompany your sales pitch. The consultation should be about exploring how to help the patient feel better both inside and out.

The Consultation Process

The consultative process begins at the first point of contact. As we mentioned in a previous section, rapport and attitude are contagious on the phone. Even if they cannot see you, people can usually tell if you are smiling. If smiling does not come naturally to you, consider putting a mirror behind the client during the consultation to remind you to do it. To lighten the mood and create connections, have a library of light stories top of mind to share about yourself, family, or staff members.

If you are a younger consultant, your personality will help you win over clients despite your youth. You would be surprised how many patients will choose a specialist they like over somebody with more experience. Many physicians find that experiencing the treatments themselves helps them sell the process better when advising patients. Sharing your own struggles with the treatment area is the gentlest and most effective way of selling. While you do this, project both a professional and relatable image.

Preparing for a successful close begins before the physician or consultant even meets the patient. A good intake form, where patients can list any concerns they may have, will assist you during consultations. Include a checklist of common concerns because the patient may not have all their questions ready. The intake form should help the physician identify the patient's primary aesthetic concerns, so all the potential treatment plans available can be shared. In other words, we want to discover their needs and offer solutions.

Put the patient at ease right away by letting them know what to expect during the consultation. Start by introducing yourself and explaining why you are there. You may want to share what is unique about your practice or your physician. Be friendly, make eye contact, and say the patient's name when greeting them. An acronym we use to help physicians mind their greeting is "TENS" which stands for Touch, Eyes, Name, and Smile. Shake their hand, make eye contact, state your name, and smile when you greet them. Many of your clients may have had insecurities about their treatment area for years but felt too intimidated to book a consultation until now. Being friendly can help your patients feel more comfortable.

Begin the consultation portion by giving a rundown of all the services you offer while assuring them you will discuss the treatment they want in detail. You should start this way for several reasons. Imagine how frustrated you would be if a patient goes somewhere else for a service they did not realize you offer. Do not assume they have reviewed your menu of services. Many patients come in with a specific treatment in mind, unaware of other, possibly more appropriate, options. During a recent consultation at a well-known medical spa, the specialist failed to review any additional treatment recommendations other than the ones I brought up. Had I known some of the other options I have since learned they offer, I would have purchased a combination of other services and spent several thousands more at that practice. The consultant should inform the patient of what services the practice offers that may address the concerns marked on the patient's intake questionnaire.

Never assume you know the patient's budget, preferences, or recovery limitations. Your job is to help patients understand what solutions are available and would create the most favorable results. Then let the patient decide for themselves. For example, the patient might not understand that multiple levels of correction and treatment exist. Our job is to start from the top and work down to where the patient feels most comfortable.

As a consultant, you are the expert. The patient looks to you to educate them on the solutions available to address their problems. As your practice grows, these small steps can be easily forgotten, impacting your sales and profitability. That is why it is important to have protocols in place and continuously train staff to follow them.

The physician's recommendation is critical to the patient's confidence in both the practice and the expected results. Since the physician is the expert, the patient expects them to affirm the best choice to create the results they are looking for. Assuming that it is, the doctor should reassure the patient with a firm recommendation before they transition the conversation back to the patient consultant with a simple, "I will leave you two to discuss the details." Try to avoid having an owner or physician present during a pricing discussion. Most people realize that it is not at the discretion of the consultant to offer discounts and will not ask without the owner or physician present. The doctor's graceful exit will also demonstrate your practice's cooperative approach to serving patients and further assure them that they are in good hands.

The patient consultant should be present from beginning to end to prevent the patient from feeling like they were handed off from one person to another. Discussing insecurities can be uncomfortable for patients even with the most skilled staff. Having someone to hold their hand throughout the consultation will smooth out the process. First-time patients may feel especially nervous and have a hard time actively listening. Some patients have waited years to even schedule a consultation about this treatment and may retain only about 10% of what the doctor tells them due to anxiety. The pre-op meeting is the best time to reinforce these details with your patient. Do not overwhelm them during the consultation.

Be prepared with several soft closing questions that help your patients visualize themselves after the surgery. This small detail will go far in raising your closing ratios. For example, you can ask about any big events they have coming up, so you can make sure they have time to recover before debuting their new look. We want the patient to picture themselves feeling confident on that vacation or at a wedding or reunion. Cosmetic elective services are a luxury–not a necessity. These procedures are often a personal and emotional purchase. The consultation is a dance, and you are the lead. Do not be afraid to guide the process. If you have asked soft questions throughout the discussion, direct closing questions prove much more effective.

Ensure your practice places the treatment plan and price in writing. Have one copy go home with the client, and put a second copy in the patient's file to stay in the office. At the consultation I mentioned earlier, I was trying to decide among three different treatment options. One of the facility's owners performed my consultation and did not provide a written price quote for the treatment we agreed on. I later called to book the procedure, assuming we would confirm pricing during check-in. Since the price we discussed was never filed, the front desk did not know what to charge me.

After I received the treatment, I was charged four times more than the price I was first quoted. After a negative experience, *"51% of customers will never do business with that company again."*[31] So you want to be careful to keep customers happy. In my own case, the practice made things right. As a courtesy, they gave me the treatment for free, and I booked the less expensive option for a future visit. This shows that even someone experienced in the industry can be confused with multiple package options available. Not only did this mix-up cause confusion for both parties, it cost the practice money. Always present treatment options and prices in writing. Having copies in two places also reduces the chance of miscommunication and helps the front desk quote the price accurately if a client calls to purchase their treatment at a later date.

31 *The $62 Billion Customer Service Scared Away (Infographic)*, NewVoiceMedia

Do not give up if the first meeting does not close with an immediate sale. The consultation does not end when the patient leaves your office. The steps you take to follow up allow you the chance to demonstrate great customer service and a genuine concern for your patients. A written thank-you note is a rarity these days, which means it will come as a pleasant surprise to your patients. I have seen this small, low-cost gesture create callbacks that often end with a successful booking.

Advanced Closing Techniques

Often I am asked to speak at trade shows on how to handle different patient types, such as the Window Shopper, the Indecisive Patient, and people new to elective surgery. The great thing about the process we teach is that it works well with almost any patient type you may come across. By asking the right questions, you can find out what they are looking for and customize your approach.

You will also find that some strategies work across the board. For example, customer types, such as a Shopper, the VIP, and the Negotiator, all respond to value-adding cross-promotions. As you conduct the consultation, be sure to mention any applicable promotions. Even better, bring up one that you did a few months ago. Then check with the front desk or a manager to see if you could offer the same pricing if the patient booked today. The promise of a deal may be enough to sway a patient on the fence. They also get to feel special while you secure a commitment. We do not recommend overusing this tactic, but it is a great tool to have for indecisive patients.

If you know what promotions you will have in the next year, you can let them know about any events coming up that may get them a better price. Many patients will not want to wait, yet will appreciate how considerate you were to let them know. Be sure to tell them about any upcoming contests in case they would like to enter. Your good customer service will keep customers happy. Never waste an opportunity to create customer loyalty.

The target market for elective surgery values extravagance. For the money they spend, they expect exceptional customer service. Millennials, for instance, *"are willing to spend the most (21% additional!) for great customer care."*[32] And consider the success of Nordstrom's Personal Shopper program. Nordstrom realized their customers desired a higher level of customer service and were willing to pay for it. Many of the department store's products could be found elsewhere and potentially cheaper. Customers come to a store like Nordstrom to be pampered by someone who knows their preferences and will go the extra mile for them.

Patients reluctant to commit will often say they are not buying because they had no idea how expensive the procedure would be, or that they need to talk it over with their spouse. In my years of doing consultations, I have found this is usually a polite excuse. The real reason may be that they did not like the staff, environment, or level of customer service they received. During the consultation, your patients screen you as much as the procedure. They can go online and know the average cost of any service or surgery with a few clicks. They show up in person to see if they want to get this service from you.

When we host events for clients, we track denials. Over an average of forty events every month, the number of patient denials for health or financial reasons has been less than 10%. If your closing ratios are under 50%, it is important to look at your customer service levels, professionalism, cleanliness of the facility, and physician communication style. We recommend reviewing the entire process from initial contact to end of consultation to spot disconnects. If you cannot find a problem, hire someone to "shop" the practice.

Successful practices close over 50% of their consultations. I have not seen true closing ratios measured over 80%. We suggest targeting a 75% closing ratio, which is a high-performing ratio. To achieve these results, you need to know the right questions to ask and master "benefit selling." A good consultant also knows that

32 *U.S. Consumers – Especially Millennials – Say Businesses Are Meeting Or Exceeding Their Service Expectations*, American Express Consumer Cards & Services

the more a patient talks, the more likely they will talk themselves into the purchase. Guide your patient through the decision tree, allow them to do most of the talking, and you will go a long way toward building a solid foundation for patient satisfaction.

Create a protocol for the physician portion of your consultation and design it to make patients feel comfortable. A surprising number of surveyed patients state that bedside manner and customer service are in the top five criteria of how they select their providers, ranking above even the physician's specialty, years of experience, where they attended medical school, and price.

While you are implementing this protocol, keep track of your progress. Do you keep a log of consultations, results, and follow-up actions? Measuring performance typically improves it. It is also important to have a benchmark of where you began to compare to where you are now. Think about the "before" and "after" pictures you take for clients to show the effectiveness of a procedure. You cannot celebrate your successes if you do not know how far you have come. At the end of this book, you will find reporting templates that you can implement right away.

In this chapter, we discussed how a well-organized consultation structure can provide the best experience for a new client and lead to higher conversion ratios. We shared some key elements to set your practice up for success:

- Give yourself enough time to educate and win the patient over, ideally with an hour-long consultation.

- If a promotion applies, mention it to promote goodwill.

- Do not assume you understand your patient's needs, budgets, or fears.

- Develop a comprehensive intake form that addresses any condition or symptoms you should discuss with a client during the meeting.

- Make sure to include a written treatment plan and price quote to prevent any confusion at booking.

Following this protocol will eliminate many of the roadblocks that prevent patients from going through with a procedure at your practice. Rise above the competition and increase profitability by applying these proven techniques to close the deal.

	1 Hour Consultation Format
15 Minutes:	The consultant builds rapport with the patient and learns about his or her concerns. They should go over all other services the patient may be unaware are offered.
15-30 Minutes:	The consultant reviews treatment options and explains what to expect. They will then step out to get the physician. They should give the physician a quick one-minute overview before they step in with the patient.
30-45 Minutes:	The physician, patient, and consultant sit down to discuss health history, medical questions, desired outcomes, and physician recommendations for the patient's treatment plan.
45-60 Minutes:	Consultant and patient review pricing, scheduling, finance, and final treatment plan, then process the deposit and set up the next appointment.

Full downloadables can be found in the Resources File at the end of the book.

ProjectedGrowth CONSULTING

1 HOUR CONSULTATION PLAN

	Action Items to Complete	Who	Due Date	Status
1	Map our your consultation format and format in writing			
2	Have a team meeting agreeing on consultation format			
3	Practice your consultation roles with the entire team			
4	Allow one hour on your schedule per consultation			
5	Train reception team on lead conversion to consultation			
6	Practice explaining the consultation process			
7	Script and practice explaining consult benefit to patients			
8	Set up weekly meetings to get consultation format in place			
9	Keep consultant in room from start to closing and payment			
10	Practice consultations with team and Provider			
11	Practice credentialing your providers!			
12	Also, practice your 30 second credentialing of yourself!			
13	What makes our practice special or unique			
14	Share your personal experiences of getting services if you can			
15	Practice building rapport and open-ended questions			
16	Use your tracking log to track consultation ratios and quantities			
17	Track closed consults per month - 70% is the goal			
18	Practice soft closing statements and transition in consultation			
19	Practice educating clients on why they should want the proper credentialed provider and the downsides of potential bad outcomes			

20	Make patient credit available during consultation			
21	Be able to offer procedure times at consultation			
22	Prepare to process deposit with a one consult close			
23	Review your benefit selling scripts for all services weekly			
24	Review and update your quote forms - new services			
25	Confirm process for office for pre-procedure and post appointment schedule			
26	Deposits at the consultation range from 50% to $500 to payment in full. Know your policy!			
27	Unclosed consultation follow up: thank you note			
28	Implement using your Incoming Call Tracker			
29	Utilize your upselling tracking spreadsheet			
30	Review results monthly and adjust process quarterly			
31	Set clear goal for number of consults per week			
32	Revise menu with all ancillary treatments: Injectables, Microneedling...			
33	List all the service to upsell, add on or bundle			
34	Be up to date on current promotions, contests and events			
35	Report of top RX skin care product sales			
36	Narrow down to best sellers and reduce overlap			
37	Review Package Bundling to create			
38	Implement Buy 2 get 1/2 off the 3rd as a standard for product sales			
39	Create full patient plan quote form for consultations			
40	Create follow up call log and turn in weekly for unclosed consults weekly			
41	Start a Patient Rewards System			
42	Implement a patient referral reward system			
43	Run monthly sales contests for staff			
	PROVEN SYSTEMS CREATE PROVEN RESULTS!			

PROFIT KILLER #8

8. HOSTING OPEN HOUSES INSTEAD OF SALES EVENTS

Open houses are a very common occurrence in the elective cosmetic industry. This chapter will explain the difference of the Sales Event compared to an open house and give you the tools to create a successful Sales Event for your practice with a strong ROI for your efforts.

A Sales Event is not your average open house or VIP night. The secret to a high-selling event is narrowing your focus and having event-only pricing. Your typical open house is an opportunity to showcase all of your services with some sort of overall discount or set packages for the event. By narrowing your event focus, hosting a group consultation about the specific treatment, and then allowing time for a physician exam, you can create a high-selling event that will affect your business positively. If planned correctly, a Sales Event will close an average of 75% of consultations or more, which can mean a six-figure outcome in one single evening. The reason? Open-house events are often visited by curious but apprehensive visitors, who are likely there for the prizes, and not too serious about scheduling a procedure. VIP events are usually big investments, and while the patients will indeed feel pampered and very important, they are not necessarily interested in scheduling procedures either. Which means the ROI will be little to none. In contrast, the Sales Event has a specific goal, a specific product, and a very specific guest list.

In our experience, many practice teams expect to produce a successful event by investing only a few hours of meetings across a one-month time frame. Of practices that allocated fewer than six weeks for event planning and preparation, 80% performed under goal, according to our PGC tracking statistics. This holds true even for well-established practices with a large e-mail list and an active social media presence. On the other hand, practices that allocate sufficient time for planning, promoting, and executing an event–

even those without existing substantial social media following or large e-mail lists–have exceeded their goals and experienced event sales of over $100,000.

We worked with a well-established Midwestern plastic and reconstructive practice that had never done a Sales Event. In the past, they struggled to organize event marketing and to create team buy-in and cooperation. Once we took them through our eight-week event program, they began to see the pieces falling into place. The practice received such an overwhelming response that attendance exceeded capacity, and they ended up hosting two events on the same day!

Event sales in this case exceeded $160,000. This is a surprising sum, given they are in an area with an unlikely demographic and the practice consists of a 50% elective and 50% insurance and reconstructive patient base. Of the thirty-three patients who attended that day's events, thirty chose to have an individual examination with the physicians. Of these, twenty-seven booked and paid procedure deposits. That is a 90% closing ratio of consultations conducted during their first Sales Events.

Their past performance benchmarks indicate that in order to book twenty-seven procedures, they would have had to conduct over fifty consultations. Most likely, these would have taken four to six months to close. Instead, they booked twenty-seven new cases in three hours. As our method yielded better results than previous sales and marketing efforts, it has now been integrated as a quarterly event in their marketing plan.

Why should you have a Sales Event?

A properly conducted Sales Event helps the financial success for any practice. Boosting revenue on a quarterly or even monthly basis allows you to stop discounting during the rest of the year.

The purpose of the Sales Event is to give each patient time to meet with the physician, to have an assessment and see pictures of their potential results, to have a private consultation to address their concerns, and to leave a deposit that commits them to having this procedure within the next three to six months.

How do you set a sales goal?

We know that if you confirm thirty RSVPs, about twenty people will actually show up on the day. Let us assume that you will close at least 50% of those twenty guests. If the average cost of your service is $2,500 and you are looking at closing a minimum of ten guests, you are shooting for a $25,000 event.

Once you have established this goal, you should set your payment expectations for the event. We recommend you require a deposit from guests to secure their event pricing that same night. A non-refundable, transferable deposit of between $500 and $1,000 has proven effective across the board.

Now it is time to share your goals with your staff. We suggest that you incentivize team efforts by setting a reward for achieving the goal. You might offer them several options from which they may choose as a team:

ATTENDEES	Goal: 30 RSVPs	Average Attendees: 20-25
SALES GOALS/ CLOSING RATIO	Goal: 50% Closing Ratio	Revenue Goal: 10 X $________
SALES	Average Case Cost?	Event Discount?

We recommend hosting one Sales Event per quarter, totaling four Sales Events per year. Write these into your Annual Marketing Plan and schedule all event dates at least eight weeks in advance of the event. This ensures you are prepared and it keeps you moving toward your goal, as well as helping your staff plan their personal calendars around your event dates.

Look at your four most popular services and decide which ones to promote and during which season. Body-focused events are great in the spring. Around New Year, we see success with "10 Years Younger" events focusing on facial surgical and non-surgical treatments. During the summer, injectable events and vaginal health events prove popular. In the fall, face or body events to prepare for the holiday season or to reverse summer exposure tend to do extremely well.

Closing ratios decrease dramatically when you widen the event focus. When clients are left to decide which area they should focus on first, they may become overwhelmed and not act or purchase at all. You can add door prizes and giveaways to gently highlight those other services you wish to promote, while still maintaining the narrow event focus that is crucial to a high-closing event.

PREPARATION	STAFF	DUE DATE
Identify 3 clear goals for your Sales Event and write them down.		
Pre-plan 4 events for the upcoming year and add them to your Annual Marketing Plan.		
Share with your staff 4 event dates and clear goals for each event.		

The Eight-Week Process

The eight-week process ensures that you will have enough time to devote to event planning, creative planning, and graphic design, while carrying out the necessary four weeks of marketing.

Eight Weeks Before the Event: Preparation Checklist

STEP 1: Appoint your Event Leader

Appoint one person to make decisions and delegate tasks as needed.

STEP 2: Narrow your focus

Identify a specific product or service on which to focus for this event. Focus on a different procedure for each quarterly event and aim to include a variety of procedures across the year.

STEP 3: Create a pricing guide

Before your staff meeting, create a pricing guide for your staff to use.

STEP 4. Schedule an event logistics meeting

Arrange a one-hour meeting with key staff members–your Event Leader and one or two other staff members in key positions who will provide valuable input.

Seven Weeks Before the Event: Staff Logistics Meeting

Before the meeting, print out the Event Checklist and fill in as much of it as you can. Fill in the rest during the planning meeting, as you and your staff discuss the topics listed below.

Event Date

In terms of attendance, Thursday is the best day to hold an event, closely followed by Wednesday and Tuesday. Avoid Monday and Friday. Make sure the event date does not coincide with your surgery day, as this may prevent you from starting the event on time. Be aware of all calendar events taking place in your vicinity that may render your key demographic unavailable, including local school schedules and vacation dates. The weeks before and after Thanksgiving and the period of December 10 through mid-January should generally be avoided. Summer vacation typically begins in May and ends in late August.

Event Time

We suggest a start time of 5:00 p.m., 5:30 p.m. or 6:00 p.m.

RSVP Goal

We have found that holding the event in your office yields the best results. Can you accommodate 20 to 25 folding chairs in a classroom setting? If your office has limited seating capacity, you might consider hosting two events back to back.

If your goal is to have twenty guests in attendance at your event, we would suggest obtaining thirty qualified RSVPs.

Sales Goal

With twenty guests in attendance, you should be able to close at least ten sales. The more thoroughly you qualify your RSVPs, the higher your closing ratio will be.

Grand Prize

If you ask your vendors to contribute, you can easily provide a prize with a perceived value of at least $1,000. Focus on services that give you a great ROI, such as low consumables or quick services.

We have found it to be extremely effective when practices offer the service they are focused on selling as a grand prize. Include the value of the grand prize on the event flyer to make the guest aware of the service's value.

Door Prizes

Door prizes entice people to attend your event, and they can be used to keep energy and excitement levels high throughout the evening.

Call your vendors and let them know that you are hosting an event. Ask them which wonderful products they would like to give you for door prizes. Look at any individual products or services you have that you would like to promote.

Reservation Fees

If you require $25 to hold a guest's reservation, then give them a gift card or credit of at least $50 at the event to be used toward purchasing a service you offer.

Refreshments

Many practices serve a fruit tray, an assortment of vegetables and cheese, and a sweet treat of some sort, and their clients are pleased. A fun and fizzy beverage is perfect for this type of event.

You can ask your vendors to help out with the refreshments. Ask them how they would like to be involved. They may wish to contribute to the cost of food and beverages or, if you are having the event catered, they might call ahead and pay the bill. If they should offer to send you a case of wine or bubbly, politely request that it arrive one week prior to your event.

Event-Only Pricing

We generally suggest offering an event-only discount of 20%. This is sizable enough to motivate the patient to sign up that same night, yet it will not hurt your bottom line. It is recommended to offer value-added cross-promotions at other times of the year and confine discounted rates to specific events only as planned.

Deposits

Set the deposit amount before the event and include it on the quotation form. We suggest setting the deposit amount at $500. Inform the patient that this deposit is non-refundable but may be transferred to a different service you provide, and that it serves to hold their event-only pricing quotation until you call and schedule them. Collect 50% of the final amount at the time they book the procedure or service as a requirement to get on the schedule.

Graphic Design and Creative Content

Discuss with your team the design of your event flyer. You can find images online on shutterstock.com or adobestock.com.

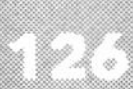

Creative content should include an eye-catching image, a campaign slogan, and several key selling benefits of the service on which the event is focused. You will want to include the date, time, and your contact information, including how you would like them to RSVP. Do not forget to tell them you will offer exclusive event-only pricing at the event!

Promotion Planner

- Headline or name and theme of the event
- Event focus (e.g., Face; Body; Feminine Health; Hair Transplantation)
- Event location, date, and time (or times, if hosting two events on the same day)
- Selling benefits for the event services (list between three and five)
- Practice info (practice name, website URL, telephone number, RSVP)
- Grand prize and door prizes
- Urgency (e.g., Limited Capacity - RSVP Today!)

Six Weeks Before the Event: Logistics

STEP 1. Create an event binder

Print and store the necessary logs, forms, call scripts, and weekly tracking sheets you will be using throughout the eight-week process. You will find these in the Resources Chapter of this book, along with links to downloadable forms.

STEP 2. Hold an all-staff meeting

Review your event plans and goals with the entire staff. Train your staff to utilize a benefit-selling method to obtain RSVPs and to accurately answer patient questions and provide valuable information in patient consultations. Make sure they understand how the new technology works and can explain its benefits to patients. Provide them with pricing structures and "before" and "after" pictures. Show them the event binder and tools you are providing and begin delegating roles to the appropriate staff members as follows:

Food & Beverage Lead

Meets with Event Leader to decide which light bites and drinks to order or purchase. Purchases and/or organizes disposable needs: plates, napkins, cups, etc. Ensures that all needed items will be on site two hours prior to event.

Table & Chair Lead

Assesses event location needs. Arranges for bulky furniture to be removed. Orders folding chairs and tables if needed and ensures that they will be on site two to four hours prior to event.

Website Specialist

Prepares content and adds to website (or coordinates with webmaster). Adds pop-up event flyer to website or to events tab.

E-mail Marketing Specialist

Creates e-mail schedule utilizing a four-week marketing calendar. Pre-loads e-mail campaigns to be sent out on Tuesdays at 10 a.m. Creates catchy subject lines.

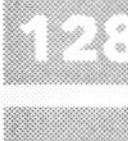

Social Media Specialist

Creates a social media marketing schedule utilizing a four-week marketing calendar.

Pre-shoots all needed videos for the campaign. Sets up and launches all social platforms during the marketing period. Responds to comments or questions on each platform as quickly as possible throughout the day.

Greeter/Floater

Attends event evening. Greets all guests at the door and assists with check-in. Creates a warm environment with guests and assumes the role of host or hostess as needed Can transition into consult facilitator and keep the energy up with door prize drawings.

Sign-In Sheet Facilitator

Keeps track of who has arrived and makes certain that everyone has signed in. Tracks who wins a prize for future follow-up. When it is time for consultations, the facilitator will manage the patient flow between the sales consultants' rooms on a first come, first served basis (in order of signing in), while also tracking all patients who have had a consultation.

Payment Coordinator

Collects deposits over the course of the event.

Sales Consultants

Provide private mini-consultation to address personal concerns of the patient. Go over pricing with the patient. Introduce the patient to the doctor making rounds between the sales consultants' rooms and then personally escort the patient back to the payment coordinator.

STEP 3. Share and edit your event checklist

Take the logistics information you created and add in the roles that you delegated. Add this to your event binder where all team members can easily access it.

STEP 4. Create excitement

Make things fun by including treats, and your staff will be more open to taking on additional tasks. If you are adding a new service, do an after-hours staff party and let them try your new procedure.

STEP 5. Discuss phone protocols and call conversion

Tell your team members how you would like them to greet the caller, how to lead the conversation with energy and efficiency, and how to convert calls to consultations or RSVPs. Having each staff member utilize a phone script will keep everyone aligned and expressing the same message. Make sure the receptionist transfers the call off the front desk to take the caller through the qualifying questions. If you must put a caller on hold, do it only once and for only a brief time. If you need to call them back, give them a time frame in which you will do so.

STEP 6. Prepare for graphic design and proofing

Gather the flyer/invitation content that you created in the *6 Weeks Before the Event* part and send it to your graphic designer or in-house marketing manager.

If your event graphics have been finalized this week, immediately start using them in-house.

Have your staff follow you on all social media platforms and make sure they are subscribed to receive your e-mails. This keeps them engaged with your event. Encourage them to forward and share posts and e-mails with friends and family.

STEP 7. Develop event presentation

Create a PowerPoint presentation to use for your consultation-in-the-round portion of the event. The main elements of your presentation are as follows:

1. Welcome and event program
2. Grand prize and door prizes
3. Service or procedure overview: Information is available from your vendors
4. "Before" and "After" photos: Use your photos or those provided by your vendors
5. What to expect pre- and post-treatment
6. Medical Q & A with physician
7. Patient and staff testimonials
8. Award grand prize
9. Event pricing structure
10. Patient private consultations

Five Weeks Before the Event: Strategic Marketing Plan

By now you have received your final graphics and event promotional materials for e-mail, website, and social media platforms. If you have never tracked your marketing campaigns, this is the time to start.

Before you start advertising, make sure that you have your new service listed on your website. Work with your website specialist to gather and create content and "before" and "after" pictures.

Do not use too many different images to create awareness about an event or promotion. Plan to use only the one graphic and use this same image and message across all your media.

Go over the best practices for websites, e-mail blasts, social media platforms, pay-per-click campaign options, and other referral sources to promote your event.

Your conversion ratio to attendees and your closing ratio at the event is the highest when you market directly to your existing patients, as well as using social media to expand your marketing efforts to reach potential new clients.

PRO TIP: *Refrain from making any other promotions for the four-week period leading up to your event and after the event.*

Four Weeks Before the Event: Promotion Game Plan

STEP 1. In-House Marketing

When your finalized graphics are delivered, begin sharing them in-house.

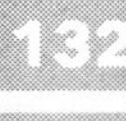

- Print large flyers, frame them, and display them at the front desk and in bathrooms and all treatment rooms.

- Order mini-flyers and place them at the front desk, on intake clipboards, and on waiting room tables.

- If your office has a monitor in the lobby running loops, or tablets or iPads with advertisements or social media links for your practice, be sure to add the event invitation and all event-related posts.

- If you have an on-hold recorded message loop, please add the event info to this loop for the four weeks leading up to the event and then delete it on the event day.

STEP 2. Digital Marketing

Here are the steps to create a successful marketing campaign for your event:

1. **Facebook/Instagram video or (even better) Facebook/ Instagram live video.** We recommend making a video with a running time of 5 to 60 seconds. Provide the date and event title and tell viewers to expect more information soon.

2. **Website:** Post a JPG of your event flyer to the Events, News or Specials tab or homepage of your website for the four weeks leading up to the event date.

3. **Event site:** You can post your event to Eventbrite free of charge, as long as you are not charging for tickets. Check which online event sites are popular in your city and pick one to list your upcoming event flyer and information.

Create a Facebook Event and post it to your Facebook Page. You can pay to promote your Facebook Event in order to widen its reach. To get the most out of your investment, target an audience living within a certain radius of your practice.

4. **E-mail marketing.** In MailChimp, Constant Contact, or your e-mail distribution system, create a subscriber list for your event campaign and upload your client e-mail list. Draft a campaign utilizing the web-ready JPG of your event flyer. Make sure to include your social media links and websites.

5. **Schedule your event e-mail campaign.** Schedule e-mails every Tuesday at 10 a.m., starting four weeks prior to your event.

6. **Make your subject lines exciting and intriguing to create a higher open rate.** Vary the way you communicate your event details week to week (e.g., event flyer JPG; video invitation; repeat flyer and mention that space is limited to create urgency to RSVP; video about service that is your event focus).

Marketing Checklist - Plan	**Staff**	**Due Date**
Event graphics approved		
Website updated with new technology and event information		
Social media marketing started		
Data-mine - Target list patients		
E-mails scheduled for delivery every Tuesday		
Video invitation posted to social media		

Event Logistics - Plan	**Staff**	**Due Date**
All staff members know event details		
Appoint someone to handle RSVP calls		
RSVP count		
Patient consultation and closing training		
Exam rooms and forms		
Set office calendar to stop seeing patients 2 to 4 hours before event		
Review and edit the event presentation		

Three Weeks Before the Event: Qualification of RSVPs for the Event

Qualification Questions:

- Have you ever had a consultation for this type of procedure before?
- Would you like to have this procedure carried out within the next six months?
- Have you researched the procedure online or elsewhere?
- What are you currently doing to address your concerns?
- Do you have a special occasion or an event deadline on the horizon?
- Do you have any questions on procedure pricing?
- Are you interested in financing options?
- Do you have Care Credit?

At this point, your prospect should be converted to the guest list for reminder calls and e-mails or moved to your next event date call list.

Two Weeks Before the Event: Boosting Marketing Strategies

Call Campaign

Create a phone script or customize one of our example scripts (found in the Event Toolkit at the end of this book) and distribute these to your staff. Allocate time for making direct outbound calls to different types of patients, as listed below.

- Target Demographic
    - Segment your patient e-mail list or your social-media targeting efforts by running a report on age, gender, client type, or unclosed consultation report via your scheduling software.
- VIP Patient
    - Compile a list of patients who are well-connected or very loyal to your practice.
- Good Candidate
    - Your staff should each be able to recommend 3 to 5 patients who would be good candidates for the procedure on which your event is focused.

In-House Competition

Engage your team members in a friendly competition to see who can secure the most deposits.

Staff Incentives

Set rewards for achieving daily goals, weekly goals, and an end goal. Some of these should be individual challenges and some should be team challenges.

Facebook and Instagram Share Contest

Invite your followers to share the flyer for the chance to win a fabulous prize. Show them the prize, describe its value, and set out the contest rules. We have found this structure to be the most effective: *1 like = 1 entry, 1 comment = 1 entry, 1 share = 2 entries*. Make a video advertising your event and incentivize your followers to share it. After the event, you can draw a name and make a post to announce the winner. We recommend doing this on video or live video! The contest winner reveal can also serve to create interest in your next event.

Facebook Boosting Ads

Step 1. On your Page, click *Promote*.

Step 2. Click *Promote Your Page*.

Step 3. Select and define your audience. We recommend targeting prospects within a 30-mile radius of your practice to maximize ROI.

Step 4. Set a daily budget to determine how much you will spend per day or set a lifetime budget to cover the entirety of the campaign.

Pay-Per-Click Campaign

We would not recommend commencing such a campaign within the eight-week structure as it can take up to twelve weeks to start cultivating leads through this method.

Marketing Checklist	Staff	Due Date	Status
What is the current RSVP count?			
Who is confirming and qualifying calls?			
Do you have seating and visuals set up?			
Food and drinks order, pick-up or delivery details			
Who will be greeting attendees?			
Who will be conducting patient consults with physician?			
Who will be collecting deposits?			
Who is printing out forms and charts?			
Who is clearing office calendar for the event?			
Create presentation for the event			
Finalize presentation and practice in event location			

One Week Before the Event: Final Preparation

Two Days Before the Event

- ☑ Confirm chairs will be delivered for the planned date and time.
- ☑ Take any pre-deposits from guests unable to make the event date.
- ☑ Prepare and practice your presentation.
- ☑ Discuss with team members the dress code for the event.
- ☑ Shop for paper goods, table linens, glassware, etc.

One Day Before the Event

- ☑ Make reminder calls or texts to all confirmed prospects (RSVPs).
- ☑ Take any pre-deposits from guests unable to make the event date.
- ☑ Confirm audio-visual equipment is working properly.
- ☑ Prepare forms: Sign-In Sheet, Entry Form, Simple Price Quote, Pricing Grid, and any handouts you may want for your event.
- ☑ Prepare marketing collateral.
- ☑ Prepare your door prizes and grand prize.

Event Morning

- ☑ Send reminder texts and e-mails to all confirmed prospects (RSVPs).

- ☑ Take any pre-deposits from guests unable to make the event date.

- ☑ Shop for flowers and refreshments.

Event Afternoon: Two hours before start time

- ☑ Make sure no patient appointments are scheduled two to four hours before event start time.

- ☑ Set up chairs, tables, food, and beverages.

- ☑ Set up and test your audio-visual presentation.

Event Evening: One hour before start time

- ☑ One hour prior to event time, have a staff meeting during which you recap each team member's key duties.

- ☑ 30 minutes prior to event time, everything should be in order. Every team member should have had a snack and look presentable in terms of hair, make-up, and clothing. All team members should be in their designated roles and ready to begin greeting guests and mingling with them.

- ☑ Take a pulse on attendance and your RSVP list.

Event Evening: Structure

- ☑ Warmly welcome your guests.
- ☑ Introduce your practice and your staff and describe their credentials.
- ☑ Give presentation or conduct consultation in the round.

Give a short presentation or conduct a consultation in the round. Describe what happens pre- and post-procedure, and what they should expect on the actual treatment day and during their recovery. Show them "before" and "after" pictures and discuss what their own results will be. Let everyone know that on this night, you will not be scheduling patients; you will collect the deposit that secures their event pricing and call them within the next few days to get them on the books.

Q&A Session

Although guests will likely ask questions during your presentation, make sure you also allocate a formal time at the end of the presentation for fielding and answering questions.

Live or Video Testimonials

Invite a few patients and staff members whom you have treated to share live testimonials during the event. Devote some time for letting them share their experiences and results with the other guests.

Draw a Name and Announce the Winner of the Grand Prize

Offer Private Mini-Consultations

Utilize your sign-in sheet and see patients in the order that they checked in. This is their one-on-one time to be assessed and signed off by the doctor. Keep it brief. If you utilize a simple price quotation form and address the patients' individual concerns, you should be able to get through about four consultations per room, per hour.

Door Prizes

During the mini-exam time, draw a name and announce a door prize winner every fifteen minutes or so. This will keep energy and excitement levels high and keep guests entertained while waiting for their own personal time with the doctor.

Deposits

Collect a $500 deposit from every guest who wants to sign up. Explain to them that this secures their event-only pricing and that it is non-refundable but can be transferred to a different service you provide. We do not recommend that you schedule patients on the night of, as this will slow things down considerably and guests may become impatient and leave. Make a copy of each quotation to file in your records.

Say goodbye to your guests, ask team members to clean up, and find a quiet corner to calculate your results. Take this away from the front desk area but complete it before leaving for the night.

Record your benchmarking statistics in the table below.

EVENT DATE:	QTY
RSVPs	
Attendees	
Consults	
Medical Denials	
Credit Denials	
Total Booked Cases	
Closing Ration	
Total Sales	
Total Holds	

Your goal is to close at least 50% of consultations held during the event. The number of patients you have declined on medical grounds or because of credit limitations should constitute no more than 10% of consultations.

How did you do? What should you do differently next time?

One Day After the Event

- ☑ Call all no-shows.
  Offer them the opportunity to come in that day or to pay a deposit over the phone.

- ☑ Close any next-day follow-up sales.
  Follow up with any guests who said they needed more time.

- ☑ Call and schedule all patients who paid a deposit at the event or prior to the event.

- ☑ Return any rentals (chairs, etc.).

Two Days After the Event

- ☑ Continue to call and schedule patients who left a deposit during event. Aim to complete this task today.
- ☑ Capture data from event sign-in form and entry forms to update your database.
- ☑ Send a handwritten thank-you card to all guests who attended.
- ☑ Add a promotional offer for guests who come back in.
- ☑ Post event pictures on social media.
- ☑ Record performance statistics for benchmarking future event goals.

PRO TIP: Along with the thank-you cards, include a promotion tailored for each patient. You can offer a combination of any services except the service you just promoted at your event.

Final Sales Event Remarks

Physicians often ask me what I would tell them after seeing hundreds of practices from the inside. The following is one of my most valuable pieces of insider information.

We hosted two events in Miami that took place in the same high-rise building a few weeks apart. Both events focused on promoting minimally invasive body contouring. The first event was held by a plastic surgery practice in their amazingly beautiful office on a high floor. The second event was hosted by a cosmetic aesthetic surgeon in a more modest office on a lower floor. They charged the same prices and set their deposits at the same amount.

You may be surprised to learn that the second event sold double the amount of the first event. Customer service and company culture are the reason for the difference. Staff members at the first practice had an air of entitlement and seemed a bit inconvenienced by their clients asking questions. They were cordial enough yet lacked the warmth and compassion that constitutes a good bedside manner. They did not seem truly happy to be working there. On the other hand, team members at the second practice were fun, warm, and customer-oriented. They seemed to enjoy hanging out and chatting with their clients. The first event sold only $30,000 while the second event sold over $100,000.

Please do not underestimate the value of a happy team, customer service, and company culture. If you are not presently offering your staff treatments and products at cost, please consider doing so. This can be categorized as a marketing expense, and it is money well spent.

Of the hundreds of practices we collaborate with every year, the ones where staff can speak from personal experience and share their excitement for this industry and their patients' outcomes are the most profitable by far. While this might sound less important than revenues and margins, a happy staff that feels well cared for has lower turnover and higher closing ratios. These offices break the industry averages.

Scaling a business is different from starting one. In order to move to the next level, you need a team you can trust to share the necessary work to create success. A valuable lesson: Take care of your team and they will take care of you!

ProjectedGrowth CONSULTING

1 HOUR SALES EVENT PLAN

	Action Items to Complete	Who	Due Date	Status
1	**Elect the Sales Event Leader!**			
2	Identify what type of event you want to plan			
3	Set up a quarterly plan for events: Body, Face, VIP...			
4	Select date for event or all events			
5	Select time - all day or p.m. event			
6	Decide on event name			
7	Grand prize			
8	Event pricing			
9	Door prizes			
10	Patient testimonials that you can ask to attend event			
11	Plan appetizers and beverages			
12	Fill out your event checklist and assign dates and responsibilities			
13	Create your RSVP Goal			
14	Create your Sales Goal for the event			
15	Event Marketing Plan:			
16	Assign these event marketing lead			
17	Select your image for graphic design			
18	Create event flyer for print quality			
19	Create event flyer for web use			
20	Create Facebook and Instagram Event Posts			
21	Create event video Invite			
22	Follow FB steps for event promotion and assign staff			

23	Have all staff added to email list			
24	Have all staff following your social media platforms			
25	Have staff call and personally invite key clients			
26	If you want to do PPC start 8-12 weeks prior			
27	Update website regarding services you are highlighting			
28	Link all event collateral to the Service Page you are highlighting			
29	Train front desk staff to take event calls and answer questions			
30	Utilize phone scripts for all staff			
31	Setup all staff event and sales training meetings			
32	Set up logistics meeting to coordinate event flow and exams			
33	Prepare patient presentation for the event			
34	Print out price quotes for the event			
35	Print our RSVP log and Sign In Sheet			
36	Prepare and print files and forms week prior to event			
37	Update your emailing list and segment			
38	Post event information in the office as well as online			
39	Invite vendors to attend and to pay for catering			
40	Ask vendors to donate door prizes			
41	Decide if you want to require an event reservation fee			
42	Have patient financing set up if applicable			
43	Stop seeing patients 3 hours prior to event			
44	Think about staffing schedule for the day - long break mid day			
45	Set up confirmation calls and or texts 2 days prior			
46	Check RSVP numbers 3 weeks prior and 2 weeks prior			
47	**If at 2 weeks pre event you have less than 10 look at options:**			
48	Active your Call campaign or move event			
49	Perhaps boosting or paid options on social platforms			
50	Confirm checklist and review it weekly with all staff!			
	PROVEN SYSTEMS CREATE PROVEN RESULTS!			

PROFIT KILLER #9

9. NOT REALIZING SOCIAL MEDIA CAN BE YOUR LOWEST COST PER LEAD

One of the most expensive mistakes you can make in any industry is to not know that social media, when used correctly, has the lowest cost per lead for marketing to your target audience and existing client base. If you gain five new clients from a social media post and the average client spends $500 for an injectable treatment, you increased sales by $2,500 from one single post. If you achieve this consistently, you are looking at an additional $10,000 a month in sales and $120,000 for the year.

You may have tried to figure out exactly how, or if, social media marketing can work for you. Perhaps, like many companies we see, you feel like you are spinning your wheels, investing countless hours without producing tangible results. In this chapter, I will discuss in further detail the key methods you should implement in your strategy and how we have used them to grow our clients' social media presence and, in turn, their revenue.

Studies show that social media followers purchase from the businesses they follow at a rate of between 1 and 5%. Based on the growth of several of our plastic surgeon clients who have grown their social media following at an average of 2,000 followers in a year, let us look at the impact it can have on revenue. If 2.5% of those 2,000 new followers purchase from the practice within a year's time, that equals fifty patients. The average patient at these plastic surgeons' practices spends approximately $5,000 a year on services. Based on fifty patients spending $5,000 a year, the practice can expect to see an increase of approximately $250,000 in revenue or sales. It is clear to see that this type of growth has a substantial impact on revenue. With the correct strategies in place, social media can and does create this ROI for many of the practices that we work with. The combination of contests on posting strategies can quickly grow your social media reach and following, resulting in increased sales for existing patients, new patients, and patient retention.

How to Grow Social Media in the Aesthetics Industry

We help our clients with social media management, among other strategies. We know what works because we do the work every day for our clients and deliver courses and lectures across the country on this topic. We started by helping a handful of clients with social media for their events. Over time, an increasing number of clients requested us to manage their social media for them. After five years of providing this valuable service, our waiting list is filled with practices needing our help. Our clients' social media follower growth averages 200% per year.

A Texas-based plastic surgeon had been running a successful practice for twenty years yet reached an impasse with the marketing strategy. They knew they needed to incorporate social media but had not had much success with it so far. They turned to us to implement three key marketing strategies–all of these "organic," which means nothing spent on ads. After building their AMP and setting monthly sales goals, we scheduled their social media editorial calendar. We created a monthly cross-promotion and a contest for each month. This in turn created the content for their weekly marketing e-mails, social posts, and written and video blogs.

Within months, the numbers began showing consistent growth. At the time of writing they had increased their revenue by 35% while gaining 2,000 new followers, which tripled their social media reach. They achieved these results while cutting other marketing costs, including print and radio. Though they spend less time on marketing than ever before, they are marketing strategically and making more money.

Creating Engaging Posts That Work

We have mentioned before that, for this industry, the critical platforms are Facebook, Instagram, and YouTube. In addition, your website, SEO, lead generation, client e-mails, monthly promotions, and quarterly Sales Events contribute significantly to your marketing ROI.

Before sharing how to create engaging posts that will grow your social media presence, I will walk you through the key terms and concepts.

Facebook algorithm: Keeping up with the content on Facebook would be impossible, so Facebook developed an algorithm to calculate which content should appear in each person's newsfeed. More than 100,000 highly personalized factors are contained within the secret algorithm, and while this ever-evolving equation remains a secret, we can put the bits and pieces Facebook has revealed to use in our content strategy.

Reach: Reach is the quantity of people who have seen your post or advertisement. Facebook will deliver your posts only to a percentage of your followers. This percentage varies according to a variety of factors, including the Facebook algorithm and advertising dollars spent.

Boost: This option allows you to pay for your post to reach more people. If you choose to boost a post, we recommend doing so in small increments ($10, $20, $30) and using targeting measures to focus delivery.

Organic reach: Organic reach describes the number of people to whom your post was delivered without boosting (paying for the post to reach more people).

Engagement: Engagement in social media can be defined as interest, which is measurable in the form of likes, reactions, comments, and shares by viewers of your content. As engagement is a significant factor within the Facebook algorithm, maintaining a high engagement rate by posting quality content will improve your Page's overall organic reach.

Certain post types are more likely to gain high levels of engagement and reach on social media. When a Facebook fan or Instagram follower comments, favors, or shares your post, they are announcing to the world that this post means something to them. You can picture it as a fishing net, and each time we cast that net wider, we are able to pull in more fish. When our followers love our content and engage and interact with it, they are helping us to cast that net even wider. Your goal is to make your followers think, *"This speaks to me."* You must find what moves your audience and motivates them to engage positively with you, thereby increasing your organic reach.

How to Share, Not Only Sell

How do we create posts that engage our audience? Take the time to ensure that every post has a purpose. People often ask us, *"Should all my posts be about our procedures, treatments, and products?"* The answer is NO!

If you are constantly selling products and services, your audience will tune out. Share varied and highly engaging content that expresses the personality of your brand, and your audience will connect with you and keep coming back for more. In this way, you build brand loyalty and nurture relationships that develop into profits when they are ready to buy.

- User-generated content on social networks has a 4.5% higher conversion rate.[33]
- 20% of people will read the text on a Page, but 80% of people will watch a video.[34]
- Studies show that people can recall 65% of the visual content that they see almost three days later.[35]

---

33 *User-Generated Content: 5 Steps to Turn Customers into Advocates*, Sprout Social.

34 *28 Fun Facts About Digital Marketing*, MySMN.com

35 45 *Visual Marketing Statistics You Should Know In 2019*, HubSpot.com.

These statistics show that original content is the most engaging and followers want to authentically get to know you and your practice. That is why we teach practices how to share and not sell.

Selling directly or by technology name does not get engagement or reach. In order to get followers excited to try treatments, you need to share the benefits and the emotional satisfaction gained by the results. This works well on social media. If you have the chance to post puppies, babies or, even better yet, videos of puppies and babies, I highly recommend doing so.

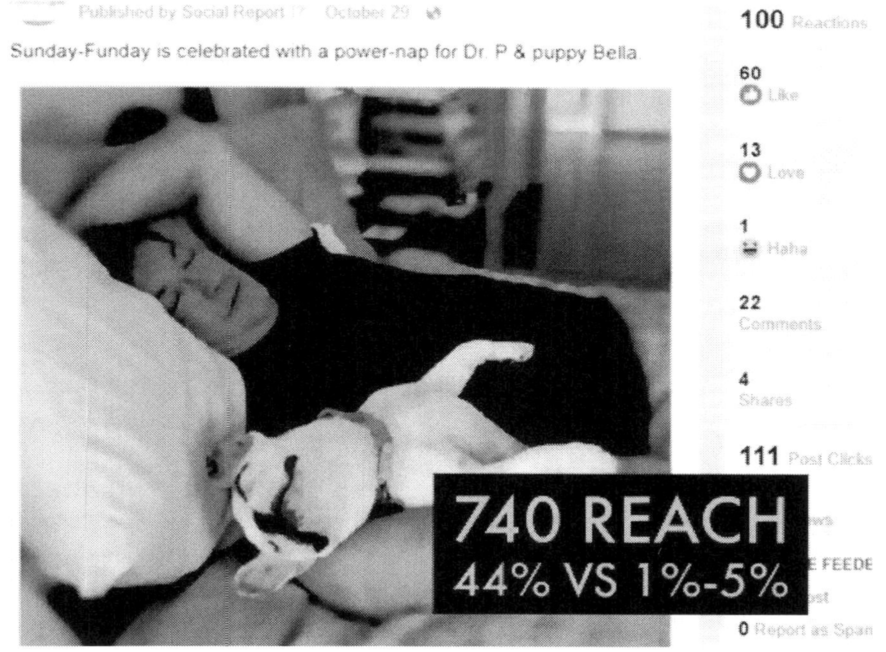

Building Your Content Strategy

> - Written articles, videos, and images are the three most engaging types of content on social media.[36]
> - 86% of consumers prefer an authentic and honest brand personality on social networks.[37]
> - 60% of small-business owners are not able to track ROI from their social media activities.[38]

Our content strategy for clients is to develop connections, provide value, and educate people about the aesthetics industry and its services, treatments, procedures, and products. The goal is to increase followers and engagement on Facebook and Instagram by building trust and maintaining top-of-mind awareness when the client is ready to seek a service or treatment. By implementing contests of the month, the goal is to create a benefit for the client for following and engaging with the practice's social media and promotions.

Create your editorial calendar a month or quarter in advance. We recommend that you post between four and seven times per week. Aim to include a variety of posts including your contest, your promotion, a fun post, a motivational post, a vlog about the products or services in the promotion or contest, sharing of office news or community news, and something showing your practice's personality or culture. Using your editorial calendar enables you to post consistently enough to really grow your following. This is the hardest part of the strategy for our clients and even for us. To ensure that your posts are eye-catching, have no more than 20% text on the image. There is no need to include your logo, practice name, or contact info because these already appear on your social media page.

---

36 *The 9 Types of Social Media Content You Need to Use,* PostPlanner.com.

37 *Brand Personality on Social Media Affects Consumer Purchase Decisions,* Smart Insights.com.

38 *Small Businesses' Social ROI Struggles Won't Stop,* eMarketer.com

As well as being consistent in posting, you should be consistent in responding to your followers. Reply to all comments, because people pay attention to your response rating and want your engagement.

We want our followers to stay engaged with us so they will purchase from us when they are ready to buy. The Facebook algorithm rewards posts with high engagement, which means you will remain more visible and be seen more frequently by your fans.

"I see you've been eating whatever you want and not exercising."
--- Pants

Things that are hard to get out of:
- Work
- Jury duty
- Sports bra

NEW MONDAY,
NEW WEEK,
NEW GOALS.

Set yourself a goal and appoint a staff member to reply to all comments up to a reasonable limit. With both Facebook and Instagram, be sure to turn on push notifications so you will be notified when fans and followers leave comments and shares.

Follow your monthly theme for the seasonal timeframe. Images are responsible for 75-90% of an ad's performance on Facebook. A recent study ran A/B testing using the same message with different images, and they performed differently.[39] When crafting the imagery for your content, take your time and be creative. Keep your target clients in mind and think about what will resonate with them.

In the following, I will walk you through the various kinds of posts you will be implementing in your editorial calendar and share some advice about how best to compose and utilize each one.

Technology benefit post

Some of your posts should highlight your procedures, treatments, and products, especially those featured in your monthly cross-promotions. Highlight the results and benefits as in the example posts below.

- Brrr! Might be a little chilly now, but swimsuit season is just around the corner, so why not ditch that razor and give us a call? We'd love to chat with you about getting summer-ready with Laser Hair Removal–the leading technology in laser hair removal! (insert your phone number) #lhr #hairfree #laserhairremoval

- Smooth curves ahead with body contouring & cellulite treatment. Confidence is sexy, so turn the volume up on your self-esteem. Consultations are free–we're ready to book yours today! (insert your phone number) #bodycontouring #cellulitetreatment #dimples #smoothskin

39 *100K Facebook Ads Tested! Here's What Works*, Consumer Acquisition.com.

Question post

To encourage your followers to comment on your posts, ask them a question.

- New Year: What are your New Year's resolutions?
- Valentine's Day: Do you believe in love at first sight?
- Spring: Where would be your ultimate spring break vacation?
- Mother's Day: Would you rather have a spa day or go to brunch?
- Summer: One piece or two?
- Halloween: What's your favorite kind of candy?
- Christmas: Do you prefer a real Christmas tree or a fake Christmas tree?

Keep it light! The question should be fun and not too personal. Get creative with this and try to make at least one question post per week. Follow the monthly theme for the season or ask a question that relates to your cross-promotion. After you have made your engaging question post and received a good response, you can then run your promotion, so it gets an excellent reach.

What's on your grill?
WHAT DO YOU WANT TO FIND IN YOUR EASTER BASKET?
TULIPS VS ROSES

GUACAMOLE
VS
SALSA

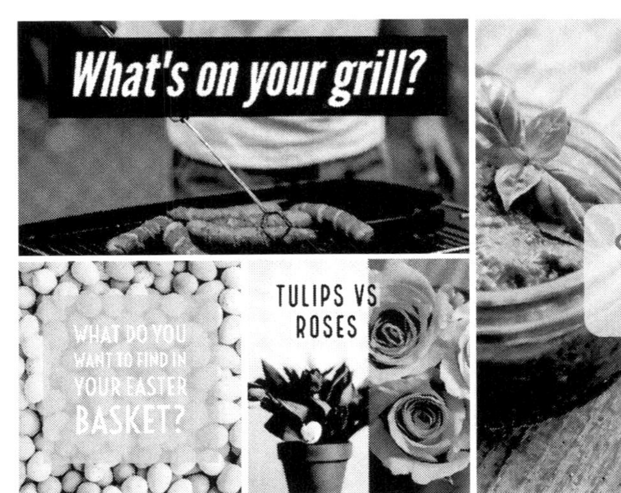

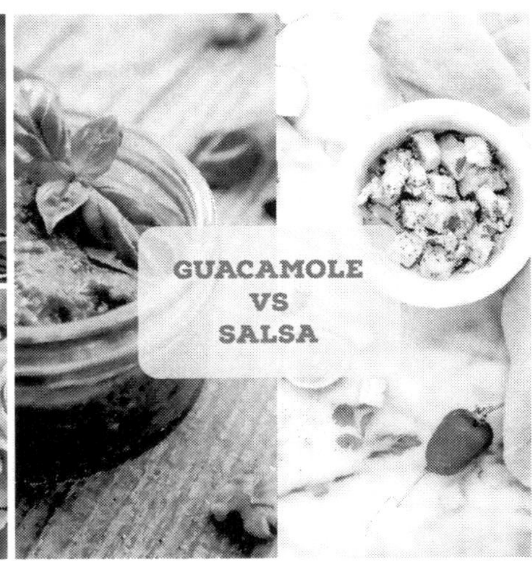

Staff highlight post

Your audience will love to see your staff on social media. Consider highlighting one staff member with weekly posts over the course of a month, perhaps starting off with a Throwback Thursday photo and revealing their name the following week. Highlight birthdays, special accomplishments, pets, babies, travel, or staff events.

We worked with a Louisiana-based medical spa that had 750 followers and needed to overhaul their social media strategy. They used our strategy to create the post below, announcing a new staff member and a cross-promotion of free brow wax with a mini-facial, and it got more than 138 engagements and 2,000 views. That is more than double their number of followers!

Renew Medical Spa
We are SUPER excited to announce the addition of Sasha Baldwin to the Renew team! Sasha is a master aesthetician with 14 years experience.
Enjoy free brow waxing and $25 mini facials through April
today for more details and to schedule your appointments!
(337) 436-3840

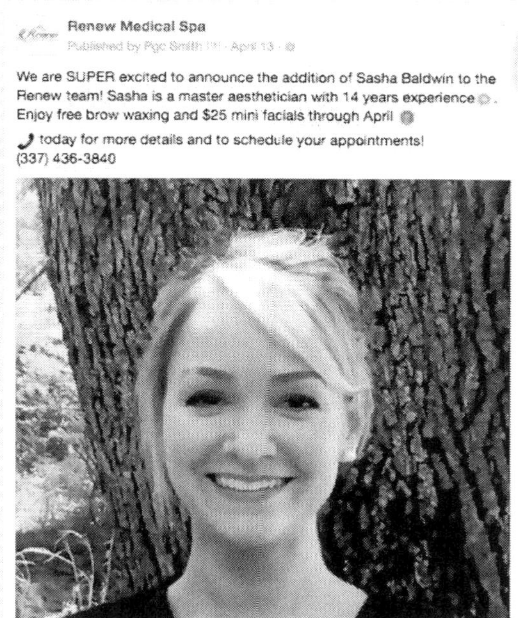

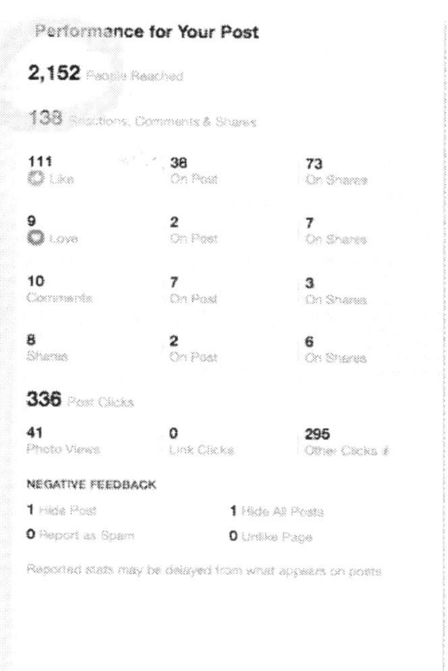

At the right-hand side of the post, you can see the results from Insights, which is Facebook's analytics dashboard. These reports show the trends, preferences, and behavior of your audience, including what they like and respond to, and you can use this information to assess the value and ROI of your social media efforts.

After implementing our strategies, this Louisiana practice continues to grow. They have cut back or eliminated all the other methods of traditional advertising that they used to carry out on a regular basis.

Posting in itself is not enough to widen your reach–you need to craft quality posts that engage your followers and track your analytics to understand and gauge the results. Doing this will help you turn likes into dollars and get a worthwhile ROI on your social media marketing.

Testimonial post

People trust their peers, so this patient-generated content is valuable. Draw on your Google reviews or patient feedback you have received on post-op paperwork, via your website, or in e-mails or greeting cards. Make your post visually appealing by including an interesting JPG image. With the patient's permission, you might take a photo of them with the physician or record a ten-second testimonial video. If a patient brings you thank-you flowers or a sweet treat, take a photo of their gift and create a highly personalized post or a Boomerang (Instagram's short videos). Make sure you have a signed photo release form from the patient.

"To earn the respect (and eventually love) of your customers, you first have to respect those customers. That is why Golden Rule behavior is embraced by most of the winning companies."

Colleen Barrett, Southwest Airlines President Emeritus

"Before" and "after" post

"Before" and "after" photos tell a story, and that is why these are one of the most popular types of posts. Include "before" and "after" photos for one of the two services in the cross-promotion of the month. When you use "before" and "after" photos, label them clearly and make sure the "after" photo is clearly distinguishable from the "before" photo. The post shown below was seen by more than 1,300 followers in their newsfeeds. Inviting followers to guess the procedure is a clever way to get them to comment on the post. Without paying to boost, this post received over 100% reach and 133 shares! Now that is a good referral campaign.

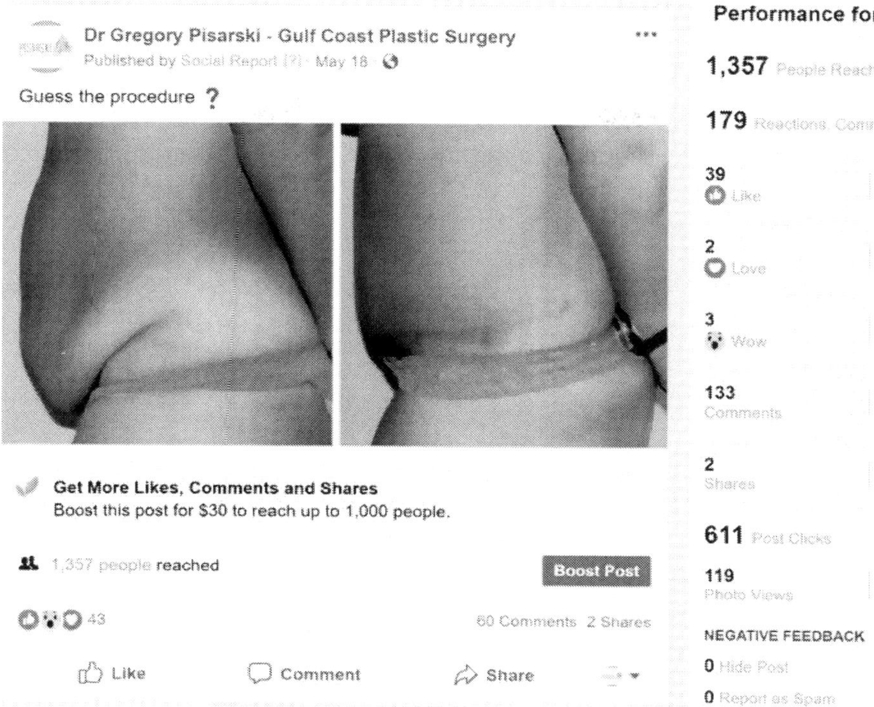
Dr Gregory Pisarski - Gulf Coast Plastic Surgery
Published by Social Report [?] · May 18 ·
Guess the procedure ?
Get More Likes, Comments and Shares
Boost this post for $30 to reach up to 1,000 people.
1,357 people reached
Boost Post
43
60 Comments 2 Shares
Like
Comment
Share
Performance fo
1,357 People Reach
179 Reactions, Com
39
Like
2
Love
3
Wow
133
Comments
2
Shares
611 Post Clicks
119
Photo Views
NEGATIVE FEEDBACK
0 Hide Post
0 Report as Spam

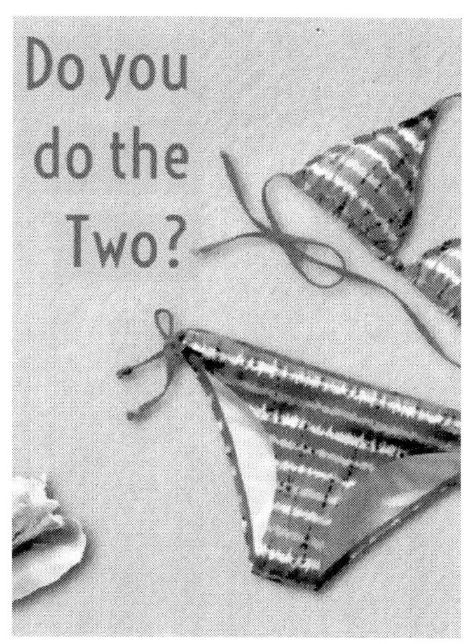
Do you
do the
Two?

Monthly Contests

Social media is all about the follower, so you need to constantly be asking yourself: *"What is in it for them? What would make someone follow a plastic surgeon, med spa or cosmetic practice?"* The monthly contest addresses these questions. We use the giveaway contest format to build awareness and keep our Facebook Page visible in the newsfeeds of our fans. As a method for gaining followers, comments, and shares, contests are more effective than any other kind of post, even those with paid boosts and advertisements.

Your contest needs to be eye-catching, preferably include a short video, and end with a question that compels followers to answer in the comments. This type of post will get more engagement and organically increase your social media reach. With the current Facebook algorithm, the organic reach on an image post is 2-6%. That means if you have 100 followers, then only between two and six people will see your post in their newsfeed.

Videos, however, triple the engagement compared to text and picture posts.[40] Video content drives higher engagement. You can see the benefit to using videos on social media. As you get more reactions to the videos, reach increases exponentially. Social media rewards the posts that resonate with the audience by sharing it more widely, thus increasing your reach. When people react to and interact with your posts, your reach increases and more eyes will see them. This is where it all starts to come together.

---

40 *How to Maximize Your Facebook Reach,* SocialMediaExaminer.com

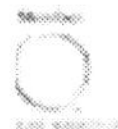

Dr. Guy Cappuccino, Plastic and Reconstructive Surgery
December 6 at 3:08pm ·

/elcome to our first contest of the month. This month's giveaway is 50 nits of Botox- a $650 value! To enter the contest: you get 1 entry for a KE, 2 entries for a LIKE and SHARE. Good luck and I hope to see you oon!

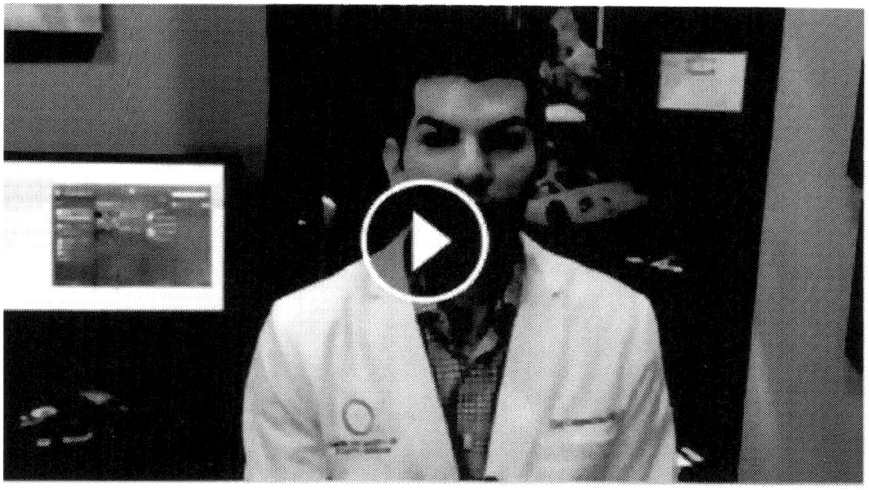

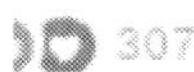

307 166 Comments 315 Shares 16K Views

I met Dr. Guy Cappuccino at a presentation I gave in Nashville. After hearing me speak about what contests can do for your social media presence, he went home and tried it out the very next day. At the time, he only had 897 followers and his best post to date had gained three shares and eight comments. Compare that to the 315 shares and 166 comments on the post as shown above. He was proud of these results, and he had every reason to be. It is not easy to get likes and shares. He posted a short video that said, "We are having our first contest of the month for free BOTOX®" and asked followers to engage with the post to enter the contest. While ideally he should have asked them to like and comment (Facebook do not allow sharing as a criteria to enter a contest), imagine his shock when this post received 16,000 views without boosting! Facebook rules change often, so pay attention to the details and keep current with regulations.

Remember, he had 897 followers. Videos get an average of 16% reach,[41] so a 35% reach for him should have been 144 people. Instead, the post reached 16,000 people. This is a 1,700% reach. This video received 166 comments and 315 shares! The Facebook algorithm identified this content as something that people were interested in seeing and pushed it out at a much higher rate. Engagement helps you get these sorts of results.

Along with consistency, asking yourself what is in it for your customer is helpful. Receiving 315 shares can be compared to receiving warm referrals from a friend to a friend. If you gave 315 patients a $100 gift card for referring a friend, you would have spent $31,500. We will not include the fact that on average, a Facebook profile has between 100 and 300 friends, and many of these "friends of friends" may have seen this post too. If we estimate that 25% of the 315 shares during the year would translate to seventy-eight new patients–and each patient spent an average of $500–the revenue would equal $43,500 in a year. Now, you tell me, is social media worth learning and doing well? After this experience, Dr. Cappuccino has a contest every month as a central part of his marketing plan.

Take a look at the post below and check out its engagement stats. This demonstrates the results you can expect by implementing this marketing strategy for your business.

By far, contests are the best way to get people to engage on social media. This post received ninety-five shares! On average, a patient referral gift should be valued at $50 to $100. The average pay-per-click lead costs $100 to $300. To receive ninety-five leads in a pay-per-click campaign would cost $9,500 at the very least, while an organic Facebook post costs only the poster's time and effort (and salary, if they are paid staff).

---

41 The State of Facebook Video In The Year 2017: Video Length Up, Time Watched Down, Business 2 Community.com

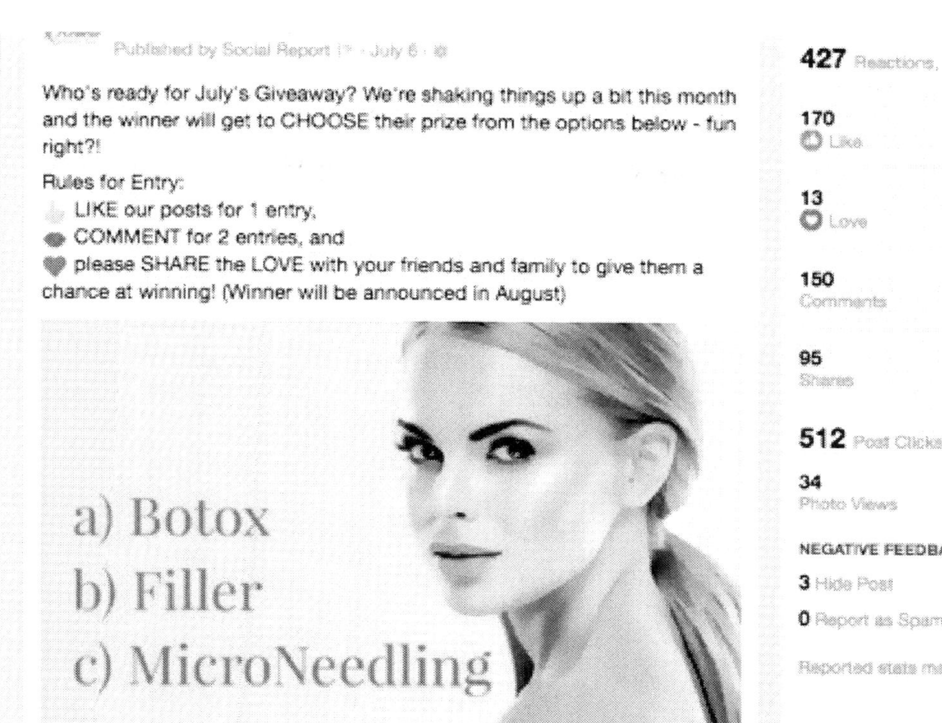

Even better, 427 patients entered the contest. They want this service, and they are your new lead list. You now have one winner and 426 people to whom you can offer a Come Back Coupon–a $50 or $100 gift card to use at their next appointment for BOTOX®, filler or microneedling. Save them to a list for an upcoming event for these services. Our advanced clients utilize these lists to grow exponentially.

The reach of the above post was over 9,000, even though the practice had fewer than 2,000 followers. That is over a 400% reach. If even 5% of those who entered the contest end up purchasing a $500 service, this post will have gained the practice twenty-one patient purchases totaling $10,500 in revenue–not to mention the value of the 9,000 people reached organically with this post.

This is how to quantify the ROI on your social media marketing. This is how you measure the success of a post. Results are analytical and measurable if you understand how to read them. Facebook's Insights reports can gauge for you what works best with your following.

Creating social media posts

Due to noise on social media, you need to catch the viewer's attention and stop their scroll, so they can see what you provide. To succeed in the current marketplace, your posts must be eye-catching, simple, and *fun*! Your posts need to make people smile, create curiosity, and make your followers *want* to comment, like, or share them. Below are a few images that have worked well for us.

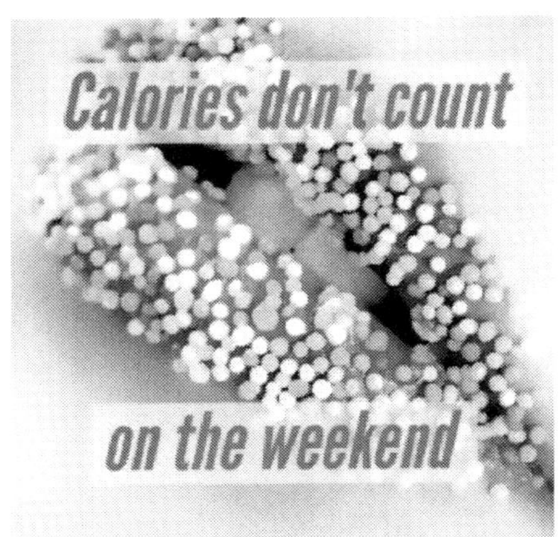

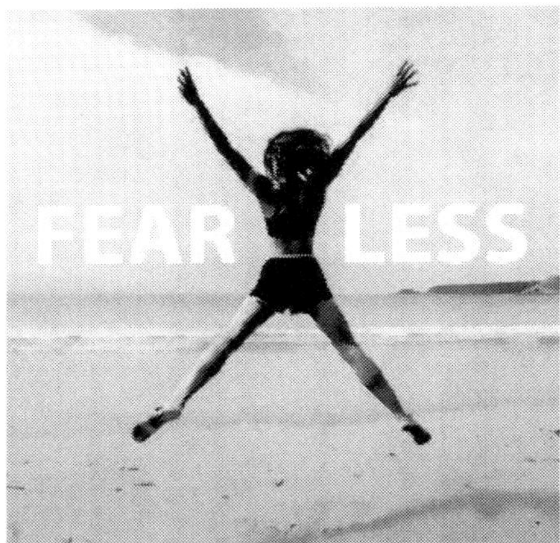

Include the details and hashtags in the captions, below the posts. Use keywords that are most often searched, so they will show up for everyone in your area seeking a solution to their problem, not only for those who type in the name of your brand or technology. Learn from your followers what works. Look at your Insights dashboard and see which content pieces your followers like and react to—and especially what they share with their friends. You can tell within thirty to sixty days what works and what does not.

Motivational, feel-good, and engagement-building posts

All of the above provide a great way to round out our editorial calendar. People find social media to be a guilty pleasure like flipping through a magazine or watching reality TV. In order to have your patients follow your social media and interact with it, you need to mix in these engagement-building posts. The goal of your social media is to maintain top-of-mind awareness among your patients, encouraging them to come back to your office when they decide they need a product or treatment. Your target market is predominantly composed of women between the ages of 19 and 64. Look at women's magazines to learn the types of things they like to read. Mix in motivation with some ways to improve and make oneself look sexier or feel better! We must speak the language of our ideal demographic. This is the time to be creative. Feminine health is a popular treatment area now. Below are some of the best-performing posts we have done to appeal to this demographic.

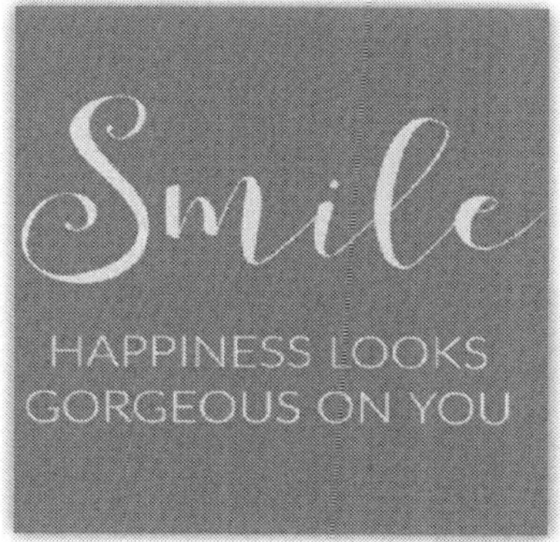

Aging is a fact of life, looking your age is not.

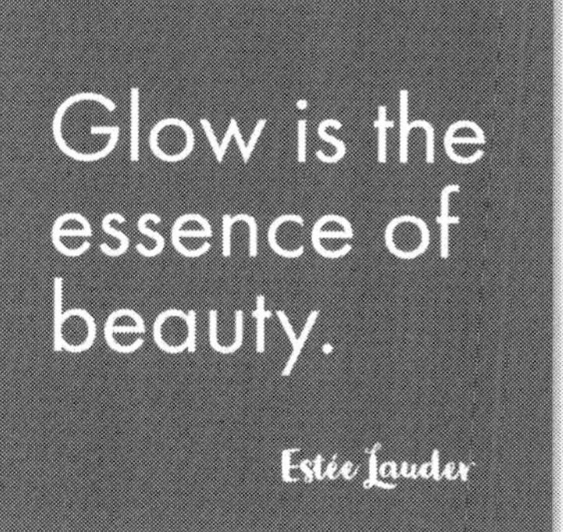

Make them smile! At the same time, make them think. This may seem obvious, but it is so often overlooked. Appeal to your target patient. Things like jumping on a trampoline or little accidents when sneezing mean something specific to your average mother of two children. She thinks, *"I want to jump on a trampoline or sneeze without worrying!"* You can communicate your message without being overt or insulting. The technical algorithmic side is only part of this formula. Have fun, be creative, and share, then fasten your seatbelts for success. This is exactly how we have used social media to attract a steady stream of new patients and grow existing ones.

Mom:
A TITLE
JUST ABOVE QUEEN

MOMS
Let's talk about our bodies after babies...

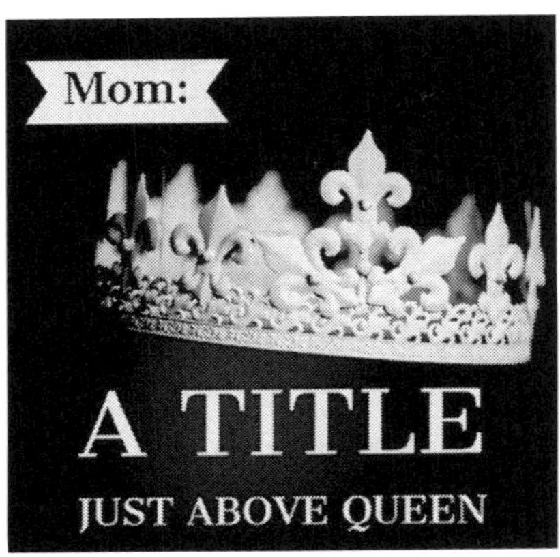

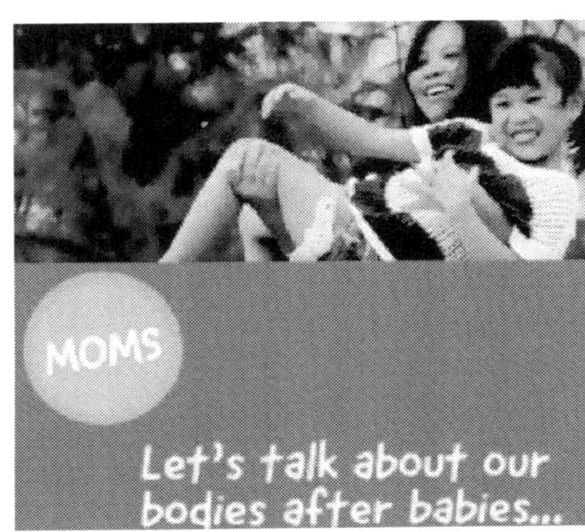

Visualizing the Post

When creating your content, consider what type of graphic and delivery will best showcase the content. For instance, if the content piece is a "before" and "after" story, would the message be better communicated via a single image, two images placed side by side, or in video format with the "before" image dissolving into the "after" image? Visualizing the post prior to designing can streamline the process for each content piece.

Graphic sizes: In social media, several different graphic sizes exist for post content, profile images, cover photos, event cover photos, and advertisements. These can differ according to the platform, and they continue to change and evolve. If you would like a current list of sizes for your graphic designer, we recommend bookmarking Sprout Social's guide, which is frequently updated.

File types: Graphics come in many different file types. For social media, you will primarily be working with JPG images. JPG is a digital raster format. The downside to JPG images is that they are non-editable and have a non-transparent background, and you cannot make them bigger without losing definition. For logos, you will want a JPG image, as well as a PNG with a transparent background for layering on top of the graphics that you design.

Stock photo resources: When designing your content, you will absolutely need stock photos to incorporate into your designs. Where do we find images to use in our designs? Can we grab them from Google searches? *Absolutely not.* Photos that you find on Google are copyrighted content, meaning they are not free for you to use. There are, however, several free resources for stock photos that are safe for you to download and use in your social media designs.

Resources for free stock images:

- Pixabay.com
- Picjumbo.com
- Unsplash.com
- Gratisography.com

Paid resources:

- Shutterstock.com
- Adobestock.com

Seasonality: Consider seasonality when you are choosing images to incorporate into your designs. Are you creating a February promotion for Free LATISSE®? Search for an image containing hearts. Is summer just around the corner? Find a great beach shot onto which you can overlay your text.

Candid photos: These always have a magical effect on boosting the engagement rate for a post because they allow the viewer to feel more connected with what makes your practice unique.

Creating Your Editorial Calendar

Now it is time to schedule your editorial posting calendar. You can use the example provided below as a guide for creating your own.

January

Sunday	Monday	Tuesday	Wednesday	Thursday	Friday	Saturday
31	1 Service Blog Giveaway Winner Post	2 FB Ad: New Likes	3 FAQ Post	4 Aesthetic Funny	5 Giveaway Post	6
7 Monthly Promo	8	9 Beauty Quote	10 Service Blog	11 Giveaway Post	12	13 FAQ Post
14 Vlog: Q&A w/ Dr	15 Holiday: MLK Day	16	17 FAQ Post	18 Service Blog	19 Giveaway Post	20 Aesthetic Funny
21	22 Service Blog	23 FAQ Post	24 Giveaway Post	25	26 Beauty Quote	27 Monthly Promo
28	29 Giveaway Post	30 Service Blog	31 FAQ Post	1	2	3
4	5					

How you create your editorial calendar is completely up to you. You may choose to have a printable hard copy and display it where everyone in the practice can access it. Google Calendar provides a great option for a shared digital editorial calendar.

Refer to your AMP. This will save hours and simplify the creation of your monthly editorial calendar for your social media platforms.

Action Items

- ☑ Create your editorial calendar
- ☑ Schedule four to seven posts a week
- ☑ What number per week is your goal?
- ☑ What types of posts will you do?
- ☑ Suggested posts
- ☑ Contest of the month
- ☑ Cross-promotion of the month
- ☑ Write blog, source images
- ☑ Write vlog script about cross-promotion products or services
- ☑ Write four engaging questions, one for each week of the month

- ☑ Feel-good posts and images
- ☑ Fun local event or news repost

Recommended Tools

Social media scheduling tools will make your day-to-day posting easier, especially if you are going to be on multiple social media platforms. You can use Social Report, Hootsuite or Sprout Social to take one post with a graphic or a video and schedule it across Facebook, Instagram, Twitter, and LinkedIn at the same time. These tools also come with reporting capabilities, so you can track your analytics to see how your social media is performing. Some also contain libraries of free images and GIFs, and a dashboard so you can comment back on all your post activity from one place.

Spark Post and **Canva** are two great apps for designing your posts. Both include a built-in free stock image library, as well as preset image sizes for various social media platforms and image types. Both applications are available in the App Store for download on your mobile phone.

Giphy: A GIF is an animated image file. They are more interactive and entertaining than photos alone. We like using the GIPHY app to search for ready-to-use GIFs to include in our posts. For example, we might search for a "congratulations" GIF to use in a giveaway winner announcement post. Another way to put GIFs to use would be to ask Facebook fans to comment on a post with a GIF. For example: *Comment below with a GIF of your favorite movie!*

Boomerang: This is a supporting app for Instagram that snaps a series of photos and edits them together in a mini-animated video. A great way to use Boomerang would be to have a new employee waving or an employee doing a happy dance for Friday. If you have a physical object to give away, use Boomerang to announce the contest by moving the product up and down.

In order to implement the suggestions to improve your social media, set up a team meeting and use the following planning guide to create your social media strategy and goals. By implementing these techniques you should see dramatic growth in sixty to ninety days.

ProjectedGrowth CONSULTING

1 HOUR SOCIAL MEDIA PLAN

	Action Items to Complete	Who	Due Date	Status
	Social Media Set-Up			
1	Designate one person to manage your social media			
2	Determine which social media platforms you will use			
3	Determine which scheduling platform you will use (example: Social Report, Sprout Social, Hootsuite)			
4	Verify that you have username & password for all platforms			
5	Verify that you have at least two staff members set in the Facebook Admin Role			
6	Create a benchmark report of your current number of followers, highest post reach, and highest post engagement			
7	Measure your annual growth prior to these changes			
8	Verify social media links are at the top of your website, and that the links are working properly			
9	Verify your contact information/address is correct on Google Maps, as well as all social media platforms			
10	Ask staff to follow you and comment on social media			
11	Encourage patients to check in and follow your social media and provide an incentive			
12	Have staff invite patients to join social media and benefits for them			
13	Create a RealSelf plan if you use it			
14	Solicit patient reviews for social media			
15	Set up a call-to-action for "Contact Us" on Facebook			
16	View your website on mobile devices			
17	Start recording short video blogs to use on social media			

18	Have a patient photo release form for social media content ready to give to patients			
19	Research and implement social content creation tools: Boomerang, Spark Post, Canva, Ripl, etc.			
	Ongoing Monthly Tasks			
20	Confirm your monthly cross-promotion and giveaway contest			
21	Create your post for the monthly cross-promotion			
22	Create your post for the monthly giveaway contest			
23	Schedule the monthly cross-promotion post once per week			
24	Schedule the monthly giveaway contest post once per week			
25	Create and schedule engaging post once per week			
26	Create and schedule a video blog or link to a written blog once per week			
27	Decide what posts you will mirror on other platforms			
28	Verify your social posts look high-quality on both desktop and mobile			
29	Utilize Facebook & Instagram Insights to track post reach and engagement			
30	Post events and specials on your website			
31	Post events and specials on social media			
32	Create video event invites to post			
33	Balance your posting types and goals			
34	Change out your cover photos regularly			
35	Track growth of followers monthly on Facebook and Instagram Insights			
36	Look at engagement and reach by post type each week			
37	Learn to duplicate similar posts that get good engagement			
38	Utilize before and after photos on social media			
39	Get patient testimonials to use for social media posts			
40	Benchmark your stats organically before you boost or pay			
41	Post job openings on social media			
	PROVEN SYSTEMS CREATE PROVEN RESULTS!			

PROFIT KILLER #10

10. LACKING A POSITIVE COMPANY CULTURE AND LEADERSHIP

It Starts at the Top

If you are anything like me, you want to find the most direct path to success. I am always looking for the most efficient approach, especially when it comes to my business and team.

I am willing to pay to learn proven strategies from the experts to ensure I will get the best results right from the outset. Tim Ferriss had me at hello. Mel Robbins (author of *The 5-Second Rule*)[42] and various other success or personal development authors and speakers share a common theme of taking action and making small incremental changes toward your goals. Business hacks, productivity shortcuts, and techniques to leverage technology and training to our benefit resonate with me on every level. This drives me to create quick and simple solutions for our clients' businesses as well as for my own.

To paraphrase Darren Hardy in *The Compound Effect*, it is incredible how much we can get done when necessary. He explains that this is because our projects tend to expand to fill as much time as we will allow. I was struck by the example he provided about how much we accomplish the day before a vacation compared to what we normally achieve in an average week.[43]

Once I found that it is possible to create an annual marketing plan with a client within a one-hour strategy session, I realized that we were spending more time than necessary to complete most of the projects required to create a profitable business.

---

42 Robbins, *The 5-Second Rule: Transform Your Life, Work and Confidence with Everyday Courage*

43 Hardy, *The Compound Effect*

What most commonly holds people back from hiring a consulting company is the fear of investing time and money without seeing tangible results. This is why our mission is to create measurable improvements and why we benchmark and track progress. Quantified value provides undeniable proof that our methods work.

Secrets to Scaling Your Business

When I decided it was time to scale my company and grow my team, I did not know how to approach it. So I sought to shorten my path by finding experts who have developed strategies for doing so. After investing in a few programs, I found the leadership and direction I needed. What I learned in the process was something I had never expected.

The road to scaling a business from seven figures to eight was not the process I imagined it to be. What has gotten you this far will not get you to where you want to be. The traits and strategies that helped you to create and start your business are not the same ones that will take you to the next level. Nor does it resemble what was done by so many of the business leaders who have become household names.

While you need to have vision, knowledge, passion, drive, perseverance, a strong work ethic, and a good business concept, all of these things put together are still not enough. When you see exactly what it takes to create a truly successful enterprise or even several of them, you cannot deny that the real underlying talent of these business leaders is the ability to recruit, build, and motivate a fantastic team that works in unison toward achieving a mutual goal.

The secret to scaling is leadership of your team. Simon Sinek, Brendon Burchard, Tony Robbins, and Brené Brown all speak about how creating a company culture of trust, safety, and win/win initiatives drives a team to mutual success because they genuinely care about each other and their clients.

How and Why Company Culture Impacts Profits

"Hiring missteps come with an expensive price tag: A bad hire can cost an employer anywhere from 1.5 to 5 times the employee's annual salary and benefits. In addition to the direct costs, indirect costs may include unhappy patients and poor employee morale."[44]

Company culture and leadership impact your numbers more than any other area. Payroll is one of your largest expenses. Meanwhile, your staffing directly impacts revenue from marketing, lead conversion, customer service, treatment satisfaction, facility condition, client retention rate, staff turnover, and your mental health. It would be terribly depressing to go into work every day if you did not enjoy the company of your team members. You are paying them to be there, after all.

If you do not like the culture of your business or company, you need to look no further than in the mirror. I did not appreciate hearing that any more than you do now. Your staff will reciprocate your treatment of them, and they will do as you do–not as you say. Trust, empathy, clarity, feedback, rewards, and corrections implemented fairly and predictably over time will grow the team you need in order to create the business you aspire to own.

We help practices define their team members' roles and clarify their visions and missions in on-site Sales Event programs. Even in programs as short as eight weeks, my team members are motivated to wow their clients and each other. By incorporating ways to wow our internal and external team members, whether virtual or local, we have created systems for expressing appreciation and gratitude, which have contributed to our profitability more than any financial strategy.

---

44 *Practice Management: Personality Testing*, MedEsthetics

"A study from modern esthetics shows that close to 70% of the doctors that own and work in medical spas are non-core. This means hiring and training the right staff to grow your esthetics business is essential to understanding the landscape of the elective medical esthetics world."[45]

Systems to Motivate and Empower Staff

Create clarity and leadership for your team by defining a corporate vision and mission, job descriptions, and high-performance management processes to generate the business growth you desire. After defining your practice vision and mission, the next step is to create the positions and job descriptions required to build your company to meet your revenue and service goals. When outlining these responsibilities, start without any particular members of staff in mind. Outline the basic job responsibilities and reporting flow, and create your company's organizational chart without any names attached.

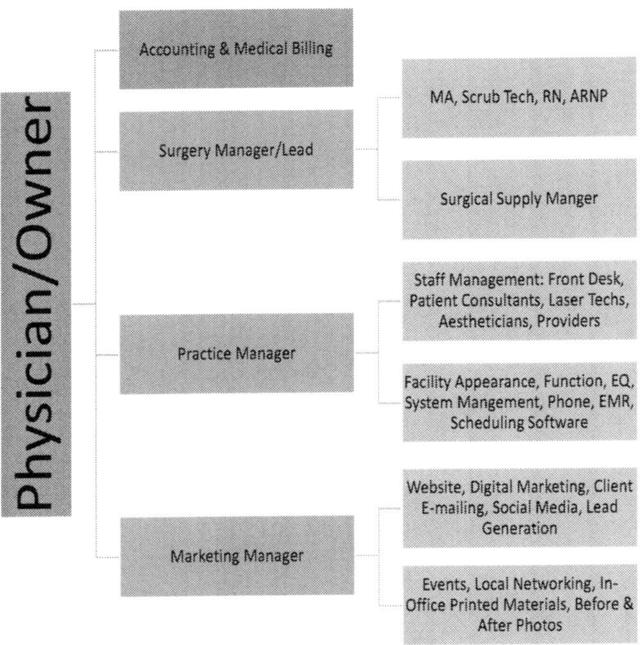

45 *"In God we trust. All others must bring data."* MedSpa Confidential, Modern Aesthetics

After you have clearly defined these positions, you can then look at your existing staff members' personalities and identify their areas of strength, weakness, potential, and risk. Match up each staff member with the position for which they are naturally suited because that is where they will thrive. You can train people to acquire new skills, but you cannot train them to acquire new personality traits. Extroverted people need to be around other people, so they do not make the best inventory managers or scrub technicians. Certain types of people prefer to work alone or in surgery.

Placing people in the positions that are right for them is the first consideration. If it is necessary to rearrange your staff, you will already know which positions you need to fill and can recruit and hire new staff accordingly. Best of all, now that you have defined the roles and their key duties and written them out, you are ready to interview and hire.

The key elements of a job description include job title, supervisor, schedule, duties, and responsibilities, as in the sample provided below. For templates, please visit us online or view the Resource Chapter of this book.

Position Title:	Medical Aesthetician
Name:	
Reports To:	
Schedule:	
Weekly Hours:	
Hourly Rate:	
Benefits:	
Commission:	
Objective:	Build rapport, educate client, set realistic expecations.

Responsibilities:	Client Care
	Treatment assessments - supporting Dr. recommendations
	Follow up after laser care by phone
	Complete charts at time of treatment
	Have patients sign consents logs
	Fill out all billing and take to front w/o client to explain to desk
	Then escort client up to front when they have freshened up for payment

Product/Service Knowledge
Participate in continuing education/consulting/trainings
Complete certifications
Attend all mandatory trainings/meeting
Research up & coming services/products (trends)

Employee Performance
Timeliness, arrive 10 minutes prior to shift
Be conscious of appointment time lengths
Stay on top of hourly schedule

Room Cleanliness
Clean room post treatments
Prep room pre treatments and clean room post treatment and day end
Monitor laundry
Abide by HIPPA requirements
Stock room with supplies
Monitor and maintain lasers, arrange repairs if needed.

Client Calls
Calling patients for events & promos
Call laser patients for results
Schedule packages all at time of payment
Run reports for patients behind on series
Turn in call log weekly to manager. Goal of five calls per shift.

Performance Benchmark Goals
See pay proposal
Repeat/request % versus new/non-request: 65%
Retention rate: 70%
Calls made per month: 20
Percent of time booked: 75%

Employee Signature: ________________
Date: ________________

Manager Signature: ________________
Date: ________________

Compensation plans define weekly sales targets, base or hourly pay, monthly bonus opportunities, salary and production projections, quarterly reviews, and growth opportunities. If you educate your staff about gross sales and net profit margins when you provide this information, they will be much more inclined to understand their production goals and the reasoning behind them.

Compensation Items	Benchmarks
Monthly Service and Retail Goals	Commission Percentage
Threshold Goals	By Profit Center
Base Pay	Hours Per Month/Value
Benefits: Vacations, Insurance, Product	Dollar Amount Value
Team Bonus	Percentage
Service Provider – Technical Level	Four Times Salary
RN, PA, DR	Seven Times Salary

When you create a strong team, the net results are incredible. Keep in mind that in this industry you do not have to hire full-time and full-benefit staff members for all positions. The benefits of products and services are a real value in recruiting and retaining your staff.

Creating your dream team begins with choosing the right people. Getting it wrong can cause immeasurable damage to your company culture, impacting morale and productivity. Add to that the measurable cost of a bad hire, which can escalate well into the thousands when you factor in compensation, recruitment expenses, and training costs. According to a recent CareerBuilder survey, companies lose an average of $14,900 for every bad hire. It happens more commonly than you might think, with 74% of employers saying they hired the wrong person for the job.[46] An article published by the Society for Human Resource Management states that it costs an estimated quarter of a million dollars to recruit and hire a new employee and, therefore, a bad

46 *How Much is that Bad Hire Costing Your Business?* CareerBuilder.com

hire can cost your company up to five times the annual salary of the person you hired.[47]

Companies without a standardized interviewing process in place are five times more likely to make a bad hire than those that do. Companies with a strong onboarding process improve new-hire retention by 82% and productivity by over 70%.[48] Aim to hire slow and fire fast. Begin by recruiting through your staff and patients. According to one article, *"Referrals from existing staff members are another valuable in-office resource when it comes to hiring… Since staff members already know how the practice runs, they will be unlikely to suggest someone who won't fit in."*[49]

Offer a bonus to any staff member who refers a candidate who is hired by you and makes it past the ninety-day trial period. The leadership of your team begins right at the start of the hiring process. You can demonstrate leadership by providing a clear structure for the journey and making it somewhat challenging to join your team. Follow this hiring protocol:

1. Résumé, cover letter, references.

2. Screening interview conducted by phone, with managers following a set list of questions to ask the applicant.

3. In-person or Skype interview with manager.

4. Working paid interview two or three hours (as a 1099).

5. Final interview with physician and other upper management team members.

---

47 *The Cost of a Bad Hire Can Be Astronomical*, SHRM.org.

48 *The True Cost of a Bad Hire*, Glassdoor.

49 Recruitment Strategies, MedEsthetics

6. Check references, social media platforms. Perform background checks, if desired. Credit check for any positions involving finances.

7. Offer letter with a ninety-day contract-to-hire period.

8. Thirty-day review pre-scheduled and dates in the letter.

9. At ninety days, convert to employee status and begin full benefits.

10. Continue quarterly reviews for first year.

11. Conduct annual reviews after first year.

Following this process will help you ascertain that it is worth the time and energy to train this new team member. They will feel motivated that they have achieved something by going through this rigorous process. Right from day one, move quickly and keep the pace fast. You cannot speed things up later if you start slow. Assign a training mentor to meet with them on a daily basis throughout the entire first month to make sure things are going well, then switch to weekly check-ins for the rest of the initial ninety-day period.

Employee turnover is costly and impacts overall morale. Create a climate of open communication so problems are immediately addressed and solved. During the first ninety days, it is important to coach up or out. Having a defined training period makes it very clear to your new hire that this is the time to prove they deserve to be part of this team and can avoid entitlement issues, which are rarely fixable.

One bad apple can spoil the batch. If you have one, get rid of it–no matter how much it scares you to do that. If it is near the top, it is an immediate priority. The staff needs to know you have a finger on the pulse and that you value the group dynamic more than one person's ego or the convenience of not dealing with the situation. A positive company culture is the only one you should accept. You are leading by example here by creating clear job descriptions, compensation plans, onboarding processes, revenue goals, weekly measurements for the staff, monthly bonuses, and, whenever necessary, corrective measures. The reward for all your hard work will be raised performance from the entire team–top to bottom.

Performance meetings and coaching sessions should be short and structured. This applies to weekly check-ins with new employees and those being coached for improvement. The main complaints from staff are a lack of clear expectations regarding daily duties, company goals, and clarity about ways to increase their income with bonuses or opportunities to be promoted. In our experience, the following format has proven most successful:

1. What are your strengths?

2. What are your weaknesses?

3. How can I help?

4. What can the company do better?

5. What can the management do better?

6. What feedback are you getting from clients?

The 1 Hour Company Culture Plan below addresses these concerns when coupled with written position and compensation plans. Once you have this basic structure in place and working, team rewards, management bonus kickers, tiered commission structures, continuing education, paid benefits, and opportunities are all highly valued employee rewards and benefits to implement.

These more advanced reward systems will instill a team mentality that creates expansive growth for your staff while protecting your bottom line.

Let us review the goals for becoming a better leader for your practice: Clarify your vision, mission, sales goals, organizational chart, position descriptions, compensation plans, and team bonus plans. Set up monthly team meetings to review goals, performance, rewards, marketing updates, patient praise and complaints, and consistent team communication. You do not have to do all of this yourself. Below is your 1 Hour Company Culture Plan to guide you in the process to a better company culture and strategy to create engaged and passionate employees to grow your practice. Schedule time with your manager or key staff members and create your action agenda and timeframe to systematically create or fine-tune the items necessary to build the team and practice of your dreams!

You deserve a big "high five" for working on your business in order to ensure success for yourself and your team. Congratulations! Remember to enjoy the journey. Because this is a marathon, celebrate the incremental accomplishments with your team along the way.

1 Hour Company Culture Plan

ProjectedGrowth CONSULTING

1 HOUR COMPANY CULTURE PLAN

	Action Items to Complete	Who	Due Date	Status
1	Create a clear vision and mission			
2	Set meeting to communicate vision, mission, and goals			
3	Create monthy staff bonus structure and goal date to implement			
4	Create timeline and goal to start your team bonus structure			
5	Create clear monthly sales goals - explain how numbers were created			
6	Set up a process up for weekly progress reports			
7	Explain the difference between revenue and profit			
8	Explain the break-even bonus structure and why			
9	Break down monthly sales goals by profit center			
10	Show goals in services per week			
11	Review average price per service			
12	Create regular monthly or weekly staff meetings			
13	Review monthly sales and next month's goals			
14	Discuss the monthly promotion and events			
15	Ask these 3 Key Questions every meeting:			
	1. How can we help you do your job better/easier?			
	2. What are our clients suggesting we do well and need to improve?			
	3. Best....I saw you do something great award!			
16	Create models to incentivize staff at an individual level			

17	Create written job descriptions for each position and staff			
18	Set up bi-monthly meetings for staff needing coaching			
19	Clarify work schedule - dates and times			
20	Review expectations for conduct and dress code			
21	Review ongoing training and meeting expectations			
22	Have staff do self assessment to compare to manager's assessment			
23	Utilize action agenda format for reviews			
24	Create fun sales contests			
25	Create employee monthly recognition programs			
26	Maintaining employee recognition ideas and events			
27	Review employee files annually			
28	Documenting corrective action - ensure this is done every time			
29	Create clear corrective action policy			
30	Update employee manual each year			
31	Annual office retreat or team building session			
32	**Clarify who is responsible for:**			
	Human Resources			
	Payroll			
	Employee handbook			
	Insurance updates			
	Staff meetings			
	Bonus program creation, rollout, management			
	Staff recognition program			
	Quarterly continuing education for all staff groups			
	PROVEN SYSTEMS CREATE PROVEN RESULTS!			

REFERENCES

REFERENCES

Aesthetic Surgery Journal, December 2018. https://academic.oup.com/asj/issue/38/12

American Express Consumer Cards & Services. "U.S. Consumers - Especially Millennials - Say Businesses Are Meeting Or Exceeding Their Service Expectations". December 15, 2017. https://about.americanexpress.com/press-release/wellactually-americans-say-customer-service-better-ever

American Society of Plastic Surgeons. "New Plastic Surgery Statistics Reveal Trends Toward Body Enhancement". March 11, 2019. https://www.plasticsurgery.org/news/press-releases/new-plastic-surgery-statistics-reveal-trends-toward-body-enhancement

American Society of Plastic Surgeons. "New Statistics Reveal the Shape of Plastic Surgery". March 1, 2018. https://www.plasticsurgery.org/news/press-releases/new-statistics-reveal-the-shape-of-plastic-surgery

Beliz, Laura. MedEsthetics. "Recruitment Strategies". https://www.medestheticsmag.com/recruitment-strategies

Bernazzani, Sophia. HubSpot. "Customer Loyalty: The Ultimate Guide". Last modified December 13, 2018. https://blog.hubspot.com/service/customer-loyalty

Bowman, Brian. Consumer Acquisition. "100K Facebook Ads Tested! Here's What Works." Last modified November 9, 2018. https://www.consumeracquisition.com/100k-facebook-ads-tested-heres-works/"

Bowman, Matt. Forbes.com. "Video Marketing: The Future of Content Marketing". February 3, 2017. https://www.forbes.com/sites/forbesagencycouncil/2017/02/03/video-marketing-the-future-of-content-marketing/#2ebed7906b53

Bucholtz, Chris. NewVoiceMedia. "The $62 Billion Customer Service Scared Away (Infographic)". May 24, 2016. https://www.newvoicemedia.com/blog/the-62-billion-customer-service-scared-away-infographic

Campbell, Kunle. Big Commerce. "29 Ecommerce Metrics & KPIs to Measure to Drive 10X Growth in 2019". https://www.bigcommerce.com/blog/ecommerce-metrics/#how-to-measure-ecommerce-success

CareerBuilder.com. "How Much is that Bad Hire Costing Your Business?" December 6, 2017. https://resources.careerbuilder.com/recruiting-solutions/how-much-is-that-bad-hire-costing-your-business

Constine, Josh. TechCrunch.com. "Facebook Hits 100M Hours of Content Watched a Day, 1B Users on Groups, 80M on Fb Lite". January 27, 2016. https://techcrunch.com/2016/01/27/facebook-grows/

eMarketer.com. "Small Businesses' Social ROI Struggles Won't Stop". June 3, 2015. https://www.emarketer.com/Article/Small-Businesses-Social-ROI-Struggles-Wont-Stop/1012559

Fagan, Laura. Salesforce. "Customer Service Stats: 55% of Consumers Would Pay More for a Better Service Experience". October 24, 2013. https://www.salesforce.com/blog/2013/10/customer-service-stats-55-of-consumers-would-pay-more-for-a-better-service-experience.html

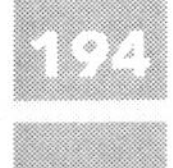

Frye, Lisa. SHRM.org. "The Cost of a Bad Hire Can Be Astronomical". May 9, 2017. https://www.shrm.org/resourcesandtools/hr-topics/employee-relations/pages/cost-of-bad-hires.aspx

Gallo, Amy. Harvard Business Review. "The Value of Keeping the Right Customers". Last modified October 29, 2014. https://hbr.org/2014/10/the-value-of-keeping-the-right-customers"

Geraghty, Shauna. Talkdesk. "7 Ways Customer Support Affects Your Bottom Line". May 15, 2014. https://www.talkdesk.com/blog/7-ways-customer-support-affects-your-bottom-line/

Glassdoor. "The True Cost of a Bad Hire". September 18, 2015. https://www.glassdoor.com/employers/blog/the-true-cost-of-a-bad-hire/

Hardy, Darren. *The Compound Effect*. New York: Vanguard, 1990.

Hilton, Lisette. The Aesthetic Channel. "Make your medspa profitable". April 9, 2018. http://www.aestheticchannel.com/practice-management/make-your-medspa-profitable?page=0,1

HubSpot. "The Ultimate List of Marketing Statistics for 2018". Last modified 2018. https://www.hubspot.com/marketing-statistics"

Hussain, Anum. HubSpot. "22 Eye-Opening Statistics About Sales E-mail Subject Lines That Affect Open Rates". Last modified 2019. https://blog.hubspot.com/sales/subject-line-stats-open-rates-slideshare"

Kruse Control Inc. "Rule of 7: How Social Media Crushes Old School Marketing". Last modified March 29, 2018. https://www.krusecontrolinc.com/rule-of-7-how-social-media-crushes-old-school-marketing/"

Leadem, Rose. Entrepreneur. "E-Mail Marketing Field Guide 2018". Last modified May 20, 2017.

https://www.entrepreneur.com/article/294536"

Lister, Mary. Wordstream. "37 Staggering Video Marketing Statistics for 2018". Last Updated March 12, 2019. https://www.wordstream.com/blog/ws/2017/03/08/video-marketing-statistics

Mangles, Carolanne. Smart Insights. "Brand Personality on Social Media Affects Consumer Purchase Decisions". July 20, 2017. https://www.smartinsights.com/social-media-marketing/social-media-strategy/brand-personality-on-social-media-affects-consumer-purchase-decisions/

Mawhinney, Jesse. HubSpot. "45 Visual Marketing Statistics You Should Know In 2019". Last modified February 5, 2019. https://blog.hubspot.com/marketing/visual-content-marketing-strategy

McEachern, Alex. Smile.io. "Repeat Customers Are Profitable And We Can Prove It!" Last modified August 10, 2018. https://blog.smile.io/repeat-customers-profitable-stats-to-prove

Medical Spa MD Blog. "Medical Spa Report: 3.6 billion US Market in 2016". https://medicalspamd.com/the-blog/2016/5/5/medical-spa-report-36-billion-us-market-in-2016.html

MySMN.com. "28 Fun Facts About Digital Marketing". March 21, 2015.
https://mysmn.com/28-fun-facts-about-digital-marketing/

O'Sullivan, Gareth. PostPlanner. "The 9 Types of Social Media Content You Need to Use". https://www.postplanner.com/blog/types-of-social-media-content

Reichheid, Fred. Bain & Company, Inc. "Prescription for cutting costs". http://www2.bain.com/Images/BB_Prescription_cutting_costs.pdf

Robbins, Mel. *The 5-Second Rule: Transform Your Life, Work and Confidence with Everyday Courage*. New York: Savio Republic, 2017.

Sarfati, Lydia. Associated Skin Care Professionals. "The Art of Recommendation", Skindeep Magazine May/June 2018, p 60-65.
http://www.ascpskindeepdigital.com/i/968907-may-june-2018/64

Saric, Marco. Business 2 Community. "The State of Facebook Video In The Year 2017: Video Length Up, Time Watched Down". May 2, 2017.
https://www.business2community.com/facebook/state-facebook-video-year-2017-video-length-time-watched-01834666

Smith, Mari. Social Media Examiner. "How to Maximize Your Facebook Reach". March 20, 2017.
https://www.socialmediaexaminer.com/how-to-maximize-facebook-reach/

Social Report Blog. Social Report. "7 Digital Marketing Trends That Will Own 2019". March 26, 2019.

https://www.socialreport.com/insights/article/360000663006-7-Digital-Marketing-Trends-That-Will-Own-2019

Sukhraj, Ramona. Impact. "14 Reasons Why You Need to Use Video Content Marketing (2019 Infographic". September 28, 2017.
https://www.impactbnd.com/blog/video-content-the-importance-of-video-marketing

Thiersch, Alex R. Modern Aesthetics. "In God we trust. All others must bring data". MedSpa Confidential. *Supplement to Modern Aesthetics Magazine* May/June 2017.
http://modernaesthetics.com/pdfs/0617_supp2.pdf

Whitman, Cheryl. MedEsthetics. "Practice Management: Personality testing". https://www.medestheticsmag.com/practice-management-personality-testing

Witham, Carrie. Industry Analyst, Inc. "70% of Buying Experiences are Based on How the Customer Feels They are Being Treated". December 4, 2017.
https://industryanalysts.com/12417_greatamerica/

York, Alex. Sprout Social. "User-Generated Content: 5 Steps to Turn Customers into Advocates". May 23, 2018.
https://sproutsocial.com/insights/user-generated-content-guide/

RESOURCES

RESOURCES

Visit

www.projectedgrowthconsulting.com/profitkillersbook

for these downloadable resources:

1 Hour Plans

- ☑ 1 Hour Revenue Plan
- ☑ 1 Hour Marketing Plan
- ☑ 1 Hour Website Plan
- ☑ 1 Hour Expense Reduction Plan
- ☑ 1 Hour KPI and ROI Plan
- ☑ 1 Hour Conversion Plan
- ☑ 1 Hour Consultation Plan
- ☑ 1 Hour Sales Event Plan
- ☑ 1 Hour Social Media Plan

Diagnostic Assessments

- ☑ Practice Diagnostic
- ☑ Marketing Diagnostic
- ☑ Website Diagnostic

Financial Tool Kit

- ☑ Client Lead Source and Marketing ROI Worksheet
- ☑ Monthly Revenue Proforma
- ☑ Weekly Revenue Tracker
- ☑ Monthly Revenue Plan vs. Performance Tool
- ☑ Expense Worksheets

Marketing Tool Kit

- ☑ Annual Marketing Plan Template
- ☑ Monthly Promotional Planner
- ☑ Promotional Graphic Design Checklist
- ☑ E-blasting Checklist

Staffing Tool Kit

- ☑ Sample Job Descriptions by Position
  - ➢ Receptionist
  - ➢ Patient Consultant
  - ➢ Master Esthetician
  - ➢ Injectable RN

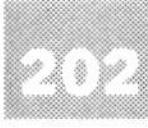

- Spa Manager

- ☑ Sample Compensation Plans by Position
  - Receptionist
  - Patient Consultant
  - Master Esthetician
  - Injectable RN
  - Spa Manager
- ☑ Recruiting and Hiring Toolkit
  - Offer Letter
  - Background Check Forms
  - Employment Application
  - New Hire Checklist
  - On Boarding Forms Kit
  - Background Check Authorization Form
  - Employment Application Example Form
  - HIPPA Sample Form
- ☑ Sample Organization Chart

Sales Training Tool Kit

- ☑ Laser Aesthetic Cross-Selling Log
- ☑ Weekly Incoming Call Tracker
- ☑ Monthly Consultations Report
- ☑ Conversion, Consult, Closing Toolkit

Event Tool Kit

- ☑ Pre-planning Questionnaire
- ☑ Four Weeks Pre-event Checklist
- ☑ Three Weeks Pre-event Checklist
- ☑ Two Weeks Pre-event Checklist
- ☑ Event Checklist
- ☑ Phone Skills and Scripts
- ☑ Best Practices for Event Marketing
- ☑ Digital Marketing Checklist
- ☑ Event Aesthetic Price Quotation
- ☑ RSVP Log
- ☑ Drawing Cards PDF
- ☑ Medical History Form
- ☑ Event Results Worksheet
- ☑ Photo and Testimonial Release Form
- ☑ Cosmetic Interest Survey
- ☑ Feminine Health Assessment Form

	ANNUAL MARKETING PLAN	
	Enter Your Monthly Promo Headline	**Promotion Value Added Cross Promotion**
EX:	*New Year, New You! .....For example*	*Free Botox with any Laser Series*
JAN		
FEB		
MAR		
APR		
MAY		
JUNE		
JULY		
AUG		
SEPT		
OCT		
NOV		
DEC		
	FaceBook Monthly Contest	Post contest on 1st, award 31st - post winner!
EX:	*New Year, New You! .....For example*	*Pick one of the cross promo items and list below - Botox or Laser*
JAN		
FEB		
MAR		
APR		
MAY		
JUNE		
JULY		
AUG		
SEPT		
OCT		
NOV		

Limited To	**Retail Value**	**Image Selection**	**Design Status**	**Promo Success**
5	*$300*	*SS #1258795*	*Final Proof*	*High, Med, Low*

Value	Graphic Template	# Entries	Winner	
$ 300.00				

ANNUAL - MONTHLY

MONTH	MONTHLY PROMOTION HEADER/TITLE	PROMOTION | VALUE
Example	New Year. New You!	FREE Botox with Laser Treatment - $250 Value
JAN		
FEB		
MAR		
APR		
MAY		
JUN		
JUL		
AUG		
SEPT		
OCT		
NOV		
DEC		

PROMOTIONAL PLANNER

IMAGE #	APPROVED ARTWORK	WEBSITE	SOCIAL MEDIA	E-BLAST	SUCCESS OF PROMO (GREAT, OK, BAD)
Face7	Yes | No	Date	Date	Dates	GREAT

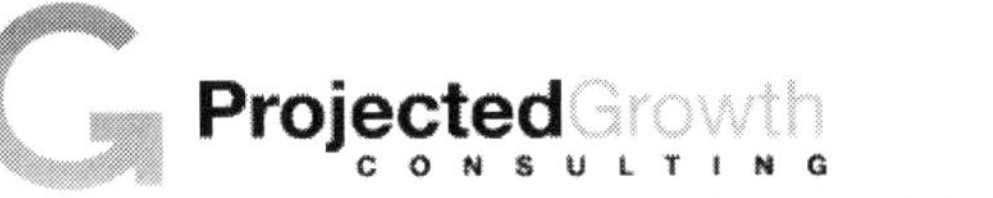

BUILDING YOUR PROMOTION CHECKLIST

1	**PROMOTION CREATION**	
	What service are you selling?	
	What season or month is the target?	
	Who is the target demo?	
	What would they like for value added?	
	Create the headline	
2	**IMAGE SELECTION**	
	Select a season appropriate image	
	Select an age appropriate image	
	Select a service appropriate image	
	Is the image attention getting?	
	Is the image what they aspire to be or your demo?	
	Is there direct eye contact?	
	Does this fit your website and marketing theme?	
	Is the image the right layout? Horizontal or vertical	
	Does the image pull you emotionally into it?	
3	**BUILDING YOUR PROMOTION**	
	Offer of cross promotion is at least 10% value	
	Value is over $100	
	Less than 3 font types	
	3 Selling benefits	
	Fun and catch headline	

	Just the details - you want them to call for more info	
	White space - make sure you have lot's	
	Review on a phone, that where it is usually viewed	
	Keep it simple and eye catching	
4	**URGENCY AND OFFER**	
	While suppplies last or first 5 clients?	
	This month only or hard dates?	
	Call for details	
	Offer not valid with other promotions	
	No cash value	
	Non transferable	
5	**PROOFING**	
	Print out the promotion for proofing	
	Have multiple people proof	
	Check website, phone, address if applicable	
	Make sure the link goes to the correct web page	
	Set up click here for consultation	

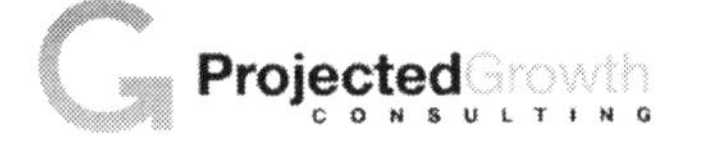

PGC Client Lead Source Benchmark Report

Revenue Total	Annual Total	Mo Ave
Current Year to Date		
Previous Year		$ -
Two Years Ago		$ -

Number of Leads per Year	Current Year to Date	Previous Year	Two Years Ago	Annual Budget Range
Organic SEO Website Inquiries				
Pay-Per-Click Leads Website				
Social Media				
RealSelf				
Physician Locator Website				
Radio				
TV				
Print				
Billboards				
Patient or Staff Referrals				
Physician Referrals				
Other				
Total				

Practice Statistics	Current Year to Date	Previous Year	Two Years Ago
Number of Consultations			
Number of Surgeries Perfomed			
Number of Injectable Appointments			
Injectable Cost for the Period			
Retail Cost of Goods for the Period			
Medical Grade Retail Sales Revenue			
Number of Aesthetic Appointments			

Social Media Statistics	Current Year to Date	Previous Year	Two Years Ago
Facebook - followers			
Facebook - Highest number of comments			
Facebook - Highest number of shares			
Facebook - Highest organic reach			
Instagram			
Patient E-Mail List			
YouTube			

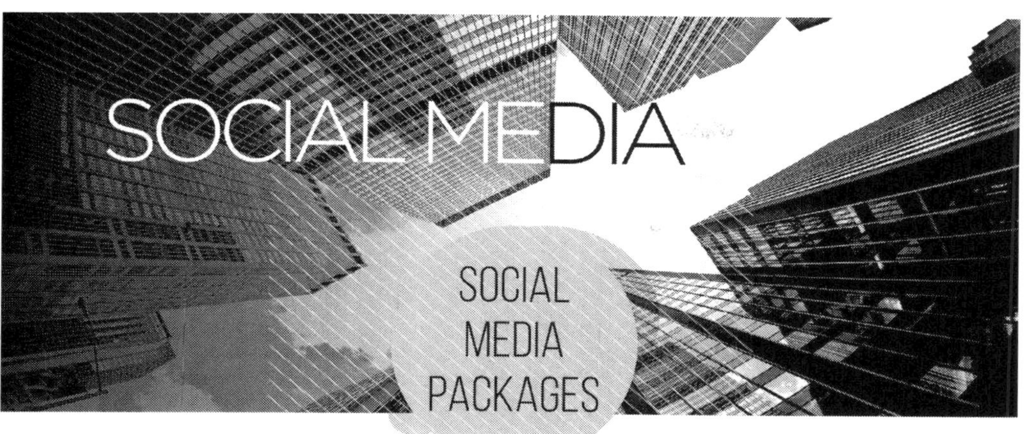

SOCIAL MEDIA PACKAGES	MONTHLY GRAPHIC SUBSCRIPTION	TRAINING COURSE	SOCIAL MEDIA MANAGEMENT	SOCIAL MEDIA MANAGEMENT PLUS
PRICE	$299 | $399	$997	$3,500	$5,000
Social Media Graphics & Posting Kit	G	G		G
Video Blogs	with $399 Pkg	G		G
12 Online Training Modules		G		G
Social Media Editorial Calendar		G		G
Contest, Event & Eblast Tips		G		G
Downloadable Toolkits		G		G
90 Day Social Media Design & Posting			G	G
Dedicated Social Media Manager			G	G
4-5 Weekly Social Media Posts			G	G
Weekly Email Marketing			G	G
Monthly Performance Review with Account Manager			G	G
Financial Benchmarking Toolkit				G
Financial Benchmarking Strategy Session				G

Kelly Smith, PGC Founder, has over 20 years industry experience, beginning with owning and operating a Washington based 7 figure Med Spa and Day Spa. She is an industry author, paid speaker for multiple laser companies, and teaches at industry tradeshows.

PGC is a National Team with proven protocols that create a high return on investment for their clients. After completing over 2,000 On Site Sales Events, PGC's experienced team will deliver measurable growth for your practice.

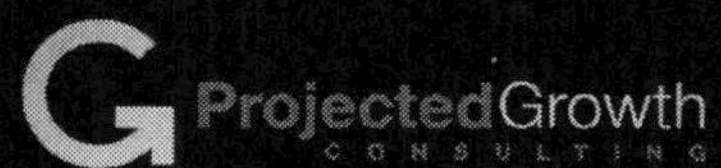

▶ 877-742-0742
ProjectedGrowthConsulting.Com

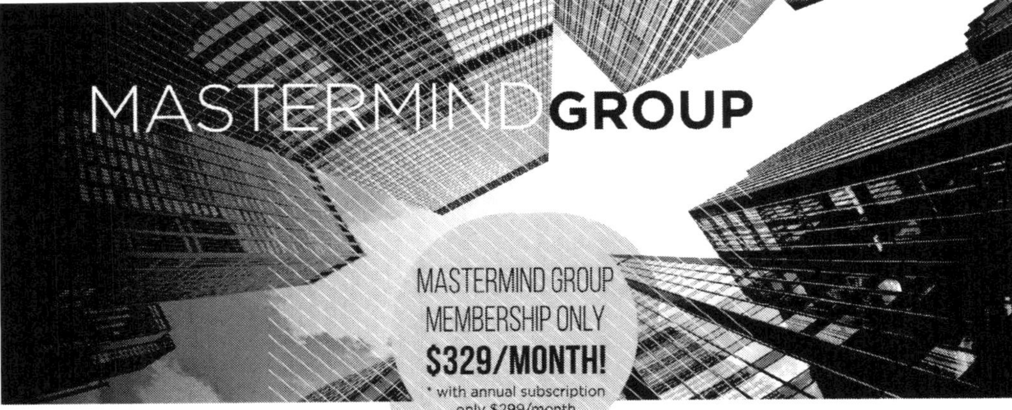

PGC has created custom training systems to elevate you above your competition. Our Mastermind bi-monthly meetings & courses will give you the competitive edge to launch your new services & increase your practice revenue.

Mastermind membership includes private LinkedIn community access:

Quarterly Social Media Digital Posting Kit

- Conversion, Consultation & Closing Course
- Annual Marketing Course
- Social Media Course
- 6 Figure Event Course

Live Webinars the 1st & 3rd Tuesday of Every Month

- 1st Tuesdays Feature Discussions on Aesthetic and Marketing Related Topics
- 3rd Tuesdays Feature Aesthetics Business Consulting with a Q & A Open Forum

All sessions will be recorded and emailed to Mastermind Members

Toolkits Included with This Program

- **Practice Diagnostic Toolkit** - Operations, Marketing, Financial, & Website Diagnostic Forms
- **Social Media Marketing Posting Kit** - 30 Day Turn Key Posting Kit for Your Selected Technology
- **Tracking Tools & Log Kit** - Tracking Logs for Conversion, Closing & Follow Up
- **Financial Benchmarking Kit** - Revenue Predictor, Monthly Goals & Marketing ROI Calculator

Additional Benefits

- Mastermind Membership in a Closed Facebook Community
- Quarterly Social Media Boosting Kit Graphics

Kelly Smith, PGC Founder, has over 20 years industry experience, beginning with owning and operating a Washington based 7 figure Med Spa and Day Spa. She is an industry author, paid speaker for multiple laser companies, and teaches at industry tradeshows.

PGC is a National Team with proven protocols that create a high return on investment for their clients. After completing over 2,000 On-site Sales Events, PGC's experienced team will deliver measurable growth for your practice.

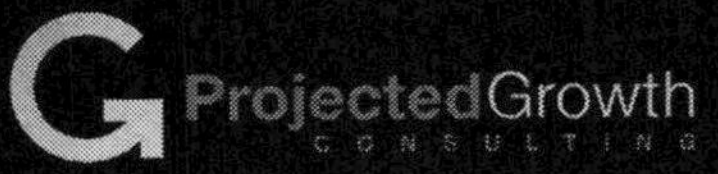

▶ 877-742-0742
ProjectedGrowthConsulting.Com

About the author

Kelly Smith is the Founder and CFO of Projected Growth Consulting and an alumna of the University of Washington. Smith has accrued over 20 years' experience as a business consultant, serial entrepreneur, medical spa owner and CFO, and was elected a 2014 VIP of the Year by Worldwide Who's Who. Alongside her semi-virtual team comprising more than 10 women, Smith continues to mentor and grow elective medical practices throughout the US.

A national keynote speaker on business success principles and an editorial contributor and faculty member for multiple industry organizations, Smith presents business and marketing practices on behalf of large laser manufacturers in the cosmetic medical industry. She is a member of Darren Hardy's exclusive High-Performance Alumni Forum and an ambassador for Women's Entrepreneurship Day in Washington and Idaho.

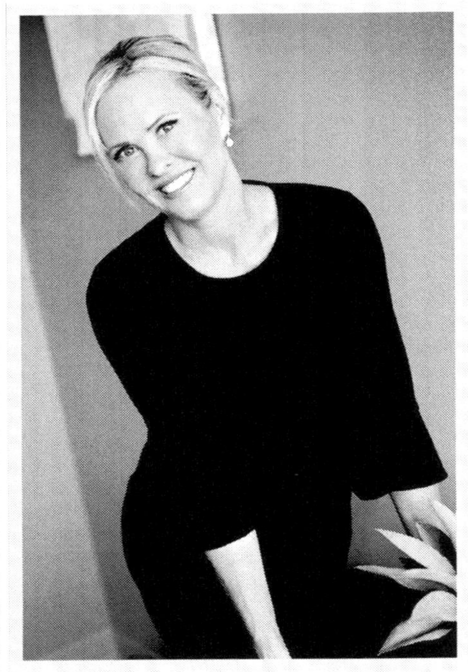

Acknowledgments

My PGC Team:

I cannot thank my team enough for building this successful company and compiling this book with me. My greatest achievement is the company culture and team we now have. This group of women makes me happy to go to work and able to face the challenges that have come over the years. I am incredibly blessed to be surrounded by such a capable, driven, and ambitious team. Special thanks to Kim Hadley, Tiffany Vakaloloma, Tanya Weiler, Nina Volostnova, Cindy Constance, Joy DeThorne, Lacey Fuentes, Kelly Sailas, Samantha Johnson, and Stacey Bernhardt. You have all gathered materials, proof-read way too many times and helped to create advice we can be proud to share with our clients and elective medical physicians wishing to grow their practices. Thank you!

I also want to mention and thank Christina Savage and Jacob Longoria for your dedication and expertise for scaling, marketing, and strategy!